Critical and Applied A
Gender a

Behavioral Science and Psychology

Series editor
Christina Richards
London, United Kingdom

This series brings together scholars from a range of disciplines who have produced work which both informs the academy and, crucially, has real-world applied implications for a variety of different professions, including psychologists; psychiatrists; psychotherapists; counsellors; medical doctors; nurses; social workers; researchers and lecturers; governmental policy advisors; non-governmental policy advisors; and peer support workers, among others. The series critically considers intersections between sexuality and gender; practice and identity; and theoretical and applied arenas – as well as questioning, where appropriate, the nature or reality of the boundaries between them.

In short, it aims to build castles in the sky we can live in – after all the view is nothing, without a place to stand.

More information about this series at
http://www.palgrave.com/series/15443

Christina Richards
Walter Pierre Bouman
Meg-John Barker
Editors

Genderqueer and Non-Binary Genders

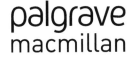
palgrave
macmillan

Editors
Christina Richards
Nottingham Center for Transgender Health
Nottingham, United Kingdom

Walter Pierre Bouman
Nottingham Center for Transgender Health
Nottingham, United Kingdom

Meg-John Barker
Psychology in the Social Sciences
The Open University Psychology in the
Social Sciences
Milton Keynes, United Kingdom

Critical and Applied Approaches in Sexuality, Gender and Identity
ISBN 978-1-137-51052-5   ISBN 978-1-137-51053-2   (eBook)
DOI 10.1057/978-1-137-51053-2

Library of Congress Control Number: 2017949533

Cover illustration: Simon M. Beer, Graphic Designer, beerbubbles.com

This Palgrave Macmillan imprint is published by Springer Nature
The registered company is Macmillan Publishers Ltd.
The registered company address is: The Campus, 4 Crinan Street, London, N1 9XW, United Kingdom

Acknowledgements

Christina's Acknowledgements

This one is for all of the kids on their own in the corner of the playground. Scuffed knees, purple bruises, and other pains less visible. The lonely; the 'strange'; and the 'weird'. For those who are 'different' or 'odd' or other, less kind, terms—maybe different in gender, maybe so in other ways.

Stay strong. You are more beautiful than you know. It's hard to understand when the world keeps beating you down, but inside of you is the fire of change that allowed us to rise up over millennia; away from the blood and terror of prehistory and towards the stars.

You see, change absolutely requires the difference which is inside of you—for if we all think the same, all act the same, we will *be* the same. With difference comes the possibility of change, and so hope, and so every last moment of progress. The difference inside of you is every revolution that felled a dictator; every cure for disease found where no one else was looking; every new word that allowed connection between separate souls; and every beautiful, profound, new idea.

As you huddle in the corner with your saviour book, or your sparkling dreams, or your talisman (they come in different forms); And the cold in your stomach twists again from the loneliness or the fear; My arm is around you, my heart is with you—and so are those of a thousand, a million, others who have been there too.

Look up. The world is waiting for us. It is awash with beauty and there is still much to do.

I'd like to take a little of your time to thank a few more people if I may? I've thanked Bornstein and Wilchins before, but it seems apposite to do so here also as it was they who first showed me back in the 90s that gender need not be a cage, but could be a pair of wings. I'd like to thank my co-editors Meg-John Barker and Walter Pierre Bouman for helping bring this project to fruition; for their deep knowledge and compassion; and for being friends I couldn't do without. I'd like to thank the authors for their incredible contributions—when I first decided upon this book it was because I lacked the knowledge contained within. I feel privileged to have played a part in bringing it together and, hopefully, moving things on a bit. Thank you also Sarah—for your keen intellect and kindness every day we work together. Naturally thanks go to my Phil for moving the whole world when needed. I'd also like to thank Margie for showing how it's possible to be smarter than anyone I know and still be gentle; Chris for somehow getting in my head with a wry grin even when he's not there—and so making me think properly, when thinking easily is too tempting. I'd like to thank both of them for being warmer, deeper, and kinder than I have any right to expect; and I'd like to thank Rio for being brighter, in all ways, than she knows; for not being afraid to be herself (an all too rare a combination these days); and not least for the joy in her eyes when I tell her the science behind what she sees on YouTube.

Walter's Acknowledgements

Walter feels forever indebted to all the people who have shared their lives, their stories, and their journeys with him in his work.

Meg-John's Acknowledgements

Meg-John would like to thank all those who have helped them in their own explorations of non-binary gender—personal, professional, and political—notably CN Lester, Christina Richards, Alex Iantaffi, Kate Bornstein, Stuart Lorimer, Andrew Yelland, Ed Lord, Jay Stewart, Dominic Davies, Ben Vincent, Sophie Gamwell, Jake Yearsley, Maz Michael, H Howitt, Arian Bloodwood, Open Barbers, and Meredith Reynolds.

Contents

Editor Biographies

Christina Richards, Msc, DCPsych, Cpsychol, MBACP (Accred.), AFBPsS is a doctor of counselling psychology and an associate fellow of the British Psychological Society (BPS). She is also an accredited psychotherapist with the British Association for Counselling and Psychotherapy (BACP). She represents the East Midlands to NHS England's Clinical Reference Group (CRG) on Gender Identity Services. She is a senior specialist psychology associate at the Nottinghamshire Healthcare NHS Trust Gender Clinic and a clinical research fellow at The University of Huddersfield. She lectures and publishes on trans, sexualities, and critical mental health, both within academia and to third sector and statutory bodies, and is a co-founder of BiUK and co-author of the *Bisexuality Report.*

She is the editor of the journal of the British Psychological Society's Division of Counselling Psychology: *Counselling Psychology Review.* Her own publications consist of various papers, reports, and book chapters, and she is the co-author of the *BPS Guidelines and Literature Review for Counselling Sexual and Gender Minority Clients*; First author of a clinical guidebook on sexuality and gender published by Sage—Richards, C., & Barker. M. (2013). *Sexuality and Gender for Mental Health Professionals: A Practical Guide.* London: Sage; First editor of the *Palgrave Handbook of the Psychology of Sexuality and Gender*; Author of Richards, C. (2017). *Trans and Sexuality—An Existentially-Informed Ethical Enquiry with Implications for Counselling Psychology* [Monograph]. London: Routledge; and is the editor of

Richards, C. (2017). *A View from the Other Side: Therapists' Art and Their Internal Worlds*. Monmouth, NJ: PCCS.
Web: christinarichards.co.uk
Twitter: @CRichardsPsych

Walter Pierre Bouman is a medical doctor, psychiatrist, sexologist, and psychotherapist specialising in gender and sexuality. Walter is the Head of Service at the Nottingham National Centre for Transgender Health. His work and therapeutic practice both focus on the area of gender, sex, and relationships, with a particular interest in the ageing population.

Walter served the World Professional Association of Transgender Health (WPATH) on the DSM-5 Consensus Committee and on the Global ICD Consensus Group. He represented the UK at the World Health Organization's (WHO) Protocol Development Meeting for Field Testing of ICD-11 Sexual Disorders and Sexuality-Related Conditions. Walter is a strong advocate for the de-stigmatisation and "de-psychiatrisation" of gender dysphoria as a classified mental disorder.

Walter serves the WPATH as the treasurer and an executive board member. He is the former deputy editor of *Sexual and Relationship Therapy—International Perspectives on Theory, Research and Practice* (2007–2016) and the current editor-in-chief of the *International Journal of Transgenderism*. He is a member of the WPATH Standard of Care Committee (SoC8).

Meg-John Barker is a writer, therapist, and activist-academic specialising in sex, gender, and relationships. Their popular books include the (anti-)self-help relationship book *Rewriting the Rules, The Secrets of Enduring Love* (with Jacqui Gabb), *Queer: A Graphic History* (with Julia Scheele), and *Enjoy Sex, How, When and If You Want To* (with Justin Hancock). Meg-John is a senior lecturer in psychology at the Open University and has published many academic books and papers on topics including non-monogamous relationships, sadomasochism, counselling, and mindfulness, as well as co-founding the journal *Psychology & Sexuality* and the activist-research organisation BiUK. They were the lead author of The Bisexuality Report—which has informed UK policy and practice around bisexuality—and are involved in similar initiatives around non-binary gender. They run many public events on sex, gender, and relationships, including Sense about Sex and Critical Sexology. Meg-John is a UKCP-accredited psychotherapist working with gender, sexually, and relationship diverse (GSRD) clients, and they blog about all these matters on http://www.rewriting-the-rules.com. Twitter: @megjohnbarker.

List of Figures

List of Tables

1

Introduction

Christina Richards, Walter Pierre Bouman, and Meg-John Barker

Introduction

This book has been hard to bring to publication. One of the first problems we came across was that the authors did not know what to write—or rather they did know, but did not know *that* they knew, as it were. "But no one's written on this before", people would say, and, in general, they were correct. There was no jumping-off point—no "Here is the literature and here is how I am adding to it", no body of work to form a firm ground from which to leap. It is notable, however, that things have changed during the time that we have been editing the book, beginning with what we believe to be the first academic conference specifically on non-binary

C. Richards (✉) • W.P. Bouman
Nottingham Center for Transgender Health, Nottingham, Nottinghamshire, UK

M.-J. Barker
The Open University, Milton Keynes, Buckinghamshire, UK

© The Author(s) 2017
C. Richards et al. (eds.), *Genderqueer and Non-Binary Genders*, Critical and Applied Approaches in Sexuality, Gender and Identity, DOI 10.1057/978-1-137-51053-2_1

gender in the Spring of 2016 (Vincent & Erikainen, 2016; see Bergman & Barker, Chap. 3) and ending with what—as far as we are aware—is the first doctorate focused entirely on non-binary experience, which was awarded at the end of 2016 to Ben Vincent (one of the organisers of the conference and a contributor to this volume). During this time, there was also a call for the first journal special issue on non-binary gender (Nursing Inquiry, 2016). Given this, and the number of postgraduate and early career researchers now studying this area, hopefully the next edition of this book will have a good deal of more specific research to draw upon from disciplines as diverse as history, musicology, media studies, law, psychology, sociology, and medicine (see also Hegarty, Ansara, & Barker, 2017).

However, given the dearth of existing literature, in some senses, the authors in this volume are the giants upon whose shoulders others may stand. But while there have been no direct antecedents to the work here, there are, of course, many whose work has informed and inflected it. The surgical techniques developed for others which have been adapted for this population; the psychological modalities adjusted to suit; and—far more so than in the other fields—the theoretical bases from which academics and theorists may work. There has been work such as Bornstein's (1994) *Gender outlaw*; Queen and Schimel's (1997) *PoMoSexuals*; Wilchins' (1997) *Read My Lips: Sexual Subversion and the End of Gender*; and Butler's (1999) *Gender Trouble*, to name a few. Note that the first three of these were from the so-called 'grey' literature—not 'properly' academic, but (as always?) beating us to it [by 20 years]. But we can go further back too from the Neolithic 'goddess' Çatalhöyük to the modern day there have been people and practices outside of the gender binary (cf. Richards, 2017), it would be foolish to assume that non-binary gender is a purely modern phenomenon and so it is to this long movement—which circles ever back to the truth from the obscuring hand of self-interested power—that this book seeks to add.

Having decided a book was needed, our main concerns were with language and the structure of the book (cf. Richards & Barker, 2015). Even the book title evolved over the time of writing as the word *genderqueer* became more accepted and utilised as another umbrella term for those outside of the gender binary—and was consequently included in the title.

One of the most difficult decisions we had to make concerned how we should entitle the surgery chapters such that readers could find what they were looking for regarding surgery for different body parts and areas, while at the same time minimising incorrect assumptions and offence. Clearly, *Surgery for Men* would be misleading and inaccurate, whereas *Surgery for Non-Binary People* would not distinguish the chapters from one another. *Surgery for People with a Penis* related gender to a single organ too closely, where we wanted to discuss a range of operative procedures—indeed, it also doesn't allow for the range of meanings people attribute to that body part. The least-worst option seemed to be *Surgery for Bodies Commonly Gendered as Male*; *Surgery for Bodies Commonly Gendered as Female*, and so on, shifting the view to the assignations of wider society, rather than our own.

This does feel like a bit of a cop-out, however. It would be nice if there were new terms, *Androsome* and *Gynesome*, say, which refer to the two common configurations of body parts developed under common genetic expression—but which do not assume a cisgender norm; and make no inference regarding meaning or gender—either of the configuration or of the individual parts. Thus, a trans man may be Gynesome, but feel his chest is incorrect and have surgery to address it. He may feel his genitals are acceptable and that, as they are his [male] genitals, they should properly be called a manhole. A non-binary person might also be Gynesome and feel that their genitals are acceptable in that they regard them as being feminine and that they fit with the degree of femininity which is suitable for them. This non-binary person may also wish to have chest surgery to effect the correct chest contour for their sense of self. Additionally, a cisgender woman might be Gynesome in that she has a vagina, ovaries, and breasts—and further she may clarify that she is content with these and views them as a signifier of her femininity, or she may seek breast augmentation surgery to effect a better chest contour for her sense of self. Thus, we split the body parts from the meaning; allow multiple meanings and options for change as required; but also have some method of communication about commonly found bodily configurations and parts which make no *a priori* assumptions. Our hope is that by the time of a second edition of this book, society, and the language it uses, will have moved so that the words we use are generally understood in this way.

We also made few allowances for readers unfamiliar with technical terms. With the Internet ready to hand—indeed with some e-readers having inline lookup functions—it feels unnecessary to continually define terms. In part, this was because we wanted the book to be technically specific, rather than being for a very general reader—although general readers should find much to interest them, and hopefully not overmuch they need to search online to define. Further, we wanted different sections of the book to be of interest to specific professions, and it feels unreasonable to ask surgeons to define simple surgical terms for the non-surgical reader when their surgical colleagues will read the chapter; or queer theory academics to do the same. Hopefully, people reading cross-discipline will enjoy the dip into another world.

The next issue concerned how best to split the book such that it has an accessible structure for all readers. We therefore decided to split it into three main sections, which nominally represented the rough areas of endeavour concerning non-binary and genderqueer folk—these being *Societies*, *Minds*, and *Bodies*. This covers the usual biopsychosocial approach to human being, but also highlights our main omission—*Spiritualities*—which will therefore be addressed in future editions as non-[gender]binary aspects of spirituality may be found in most major religions and a vast number of spiritual practices (cf. Richards, 2014). Therefore, the sections of the book are as follows:

In the *Societies* section, S. Bear Bergman and Meg-John Barker wrote on *Activism* and its place in moving the whole field forward; Ben Vincent and Ana Manzano-Santaella wrote about *History and Cultural Diversity*, giving an excellent overview of how gender has been understood across time and space in a way which alerts us to the unusual status of the current high GDP Western understanding of gender as a binary opposite; Rob Clucas and Stephen Whittle detail the current legal position in *Law*; and Jay Stewart eloquently explains *Academic Theory* in this area. In the *Minds* section, we, as editors and colleagues, each took our specialty, with Meg-John Barker and Alex Iantaffi exploring *Psychotherapy* with non-binary people; Christina Richards meditating on the philosophy and practice of *Psychology*; and Sarah Murjan and Walter Pierre Bouman giving a thoughtful overview of *Psychiatry*. In the *Bodies* section, Leighton Seal explains what may and may not be done in *Adult Endocrinology*;

with Gary Butler similarly detailing this for *Child Endocrinology*. James Bellringer explains what genital surgical options are available in *Surgery for Bodies Commonly Gendered as Male*; David Ralph, Nim Christopher, and Giulio Garaffa similarly examine genital surgical options in *Surgery for Bodies Commonly Gendered as Female*; Andrew Yelland then explains surgical possibilities in *Breast Surgery*; and finally, Alex Iantaffi considers where we might go from here in *Future Directions*.

Non-binary People: Who Are We Talking About?

Who then are we talking about when we consider non-binary people? And how many non-binary people are there? Essentially, of course, genderqueer or non-binary people are simply people who are not male or female; but as ever things are more complex than that. In general, non-binary or genderqueer refers to people's identity, rather than physicality at birth; but it does not exclude people who are intersex or have a diversity/disorder of sexual development who also identify in this way. Whatever their birth physicality, there are non-binary people who identify as a single fixed gender position other than male or female. There are those who have a fluid gender. There are those who have no gender. And there are those who disagree with the very idea of gender. You will find out more about all of these groups in the chapters to come.

It follows from this—and from the fact that most research still only offers binary choices for gender—that the proportion of the general population who are non-binary is very difficult to measure. For example, one recent review of the UK literature in this area defined non-binary as "An umbrella term for any gender (or lack of gender) that would not be adequately represented by an either/or choice between 'man' or 'woman'" (Titman, 2014). Under this definition, Titman reported that at least 0.4% of the UK population defines as non-binary when given a three-way choice in terms of female, male, or another description; and indeed around a quarter to a third of trans people identify in some way outside the binary.

Another study found that around 5% of young LGBT people identify as something other than male or female (METRO Youth Chances,

2014), suggesting that identifying in this way may be becoming more common among younger populations. In the United States, the *Injustice at Every Turn* research, which included responses from over 6000 transgender people, found that 13% of respondents chose the option "A gender not listed here" and 860 of those respondents wrote in their own gender identity terms (Harrison, Grant, & Herman, 2012).

It is clear that more and more people are identifying and making sense of their experience in these kinds of ways now that non-binary understandings of gender are more readily available through online resources and communities; through options on social media (Barker, 2014); and through visible articles and celebrities in mainstream media (e.g. Brisbane, 2015; Ford, 2015). Therefore, the proportion of people identifying with non-binary gender is constantly shifting and almost impossible to measure accurately.

Another issue which makes measurement very difficult, and which is important to be mindful of in professional practice—of whatever sort—is that whilst relatively few people may *identify* as non-binary (to the point of using a non-binary gender label or refusing to tick the 'male/female' box on a form), many more people *experience* themselves in non-binary ways. Indeed, Joel, Tarrasch, Berman, Mukamel, and Ziv (2013) found that over a third of people in the general population felt to some extent that they were the 'other' gender, both genders, and/or neither gender. These are not small numbers, and it therefore behoves professionals from all walks of life to educate themselves to a basic extent, and not to assume that the people whom this book concerns are a 'niche' population.

Instead, it is important to recognise that, whatever its numbers, this population has been around for a very long time—if only now coming to the [high GDP global Western] public eye. Consequently, non-binary folk are entitled to full legal protections and such surgical; endocrinological, and psychological assistance as might be required. Communities should be supported and not exploited. And, as ever, when our theories, training, and culture fail; we might raise our gaze a little and look to respect and kindness to guide us as they seldom lead us wrong. Hopefully, this book contains a little of all of these things and will assist in fostering more.

References

Barker, M. (2014, February 15). *57 Genders (and None for Me)? Reflections on the New Facebook Gender Categories.* Rewriting the Rules. Retrieved June 13, 2014, from http://www.rewritingtherules.wordpress.com/2014/02/15/57-genders-and-none-for-me-reflections-on-the-new-facebook-gender-categories

Brisbane, L. (2015, June 22). Why Miley Cyrus and Ruby Rose are Embracing 'Gender Fluidity'. *The Evening Standard.* Retrieved August 10, 2015, from http://www.standard.co.uk/lifestyle/london-life/why-miley-cyrus-and-ruby-rose-are-embracing-gender-fluidity-10335949.html

Bornstein, K. (1994). *Gender Outlaw.* London: Routledge.

Butler, J. (1999). *Gender Trouble.* New York: Routledge.

Ford, T. (2015, August 7). My Life Without Gender. *The Guardian.* Retrieved August 10, 2015, from http://www.theguardian.com/world/2015/aug/07/my-life-without-gender-strangers-are-desperate-to-know-what-genitalia-i-have

Harrison, J., Grant, J., & Herman, J. L. (2012). *A Gender Not Listed Here: Genderqueers, Gender Rebels, and Otherwise in the National Transgender Discrimination Survey.* Los Angeles: eScholarship, University of California.

Hegarty, P., Ansara, G., & Barker, M.-J. (2017). Non-Binary Gender Identities. In N. Dess, J. Marecek, D. Best, & L. Bell (Eds.), *Psychology of Gender, Sex, and Sexualities.* Oxford: Oxford University Press.

Joel, D., Tarrasch, R., Berman, Z., Mukamel, M., & Ziv, E. (2013). Queering Gender: Studying Gender Identity in 'Normative' Individuals. *Psychology & Sexuality, 5*(4), 291–321.

Queen, C., & Schimel, L. (Eds.). (1997). *PoMoSexuals.* San Francisco: Cleis Press.

Richards, C. (2014). *Third Genders. The Wiley-Blackwell Encyclopedia of Gender and Sexuality Studies.* Hoboken, NJ: Wiley-Blackwell.

Richards, C. (2017). *Trans and Sexuality—An existentially-Informed Ethical Enquiry with Implications for Counselling Psychology* [Monograph]. London: Routledge.

Richards, C., & Barker, M. J. (2015). Introduction. In C. Richards & M. J. Barker (Eds.), *The Palgrave Handbook of the Psychology of Sexuality and Gender* (pp. 1–4). London: Palgrave Macmillan.

Titman, N. (2014). How Many People in the United Kingdom are Nonbinary? Retrieved August 10, 2015, from http://www.practicalandrogyny.com/2014/12/16/how-many-people-in-the-uk-are-nonbinary

Vincent, B., & Erikainen, S. (2016, March 22). *Moving Beyond the Binaries Of Sex And Gender: Non-Binary Identities, Bodies, and Discourses.* University of Leeds Conference. Conference Booklet. Retrieved from http://www.gires. org.uk/pdfs/Conference%20Booklet.pdf
Wilchins, R. A. (1997). *Read My Lips: Sexual Subversion and the End of Gender.* Ann Arbor, MI: Firebrand Books.

Further Reading

Bornstein, K. (1994). *Gender Outlaw.* London: Routledge.
Bornstein, K., & Bergman, S. B. (Eds.). (2010). *Gender Outlaws: The Next Generation.* New York: Avalon Publishing Group.
Butler, J. (1999). *Gender Trouble.* New York: Routledge.
Barker, M. J., & Richards, C. (2015). Further Genders. In C. Richards & M. Barker (Eds.), *Handbook of the Psychology of Sexuality and Gender* (pp. 166–182). Basingstoke: Palgrave Macmillan.
Queen, C., & Schimel, L. (Eds.). (1997). *PoMoSexuals.* San Francisco: Cleis Press.
Richards, C., Bouman, W. P., Seal, L., Barker, M. J., Nieder, T., & T'Sjoen, G. (2016). Non-binary or Genderqueer Genders. *International Review of Psychiatry, 28*(1), 95–102.
Wilchins, R. A. (1997). *Read My Lips: Sexual Subversion and the End of Gender.* Ann Arbor, MI: Firebrand Books.

Part I

Societies

2

History and Cultural Diversity

Ben Vincent and Ana Manzano

Introduction

Only hundreds of years ago, gender was not commonly or instinctively binarised. This chapter explores multiple understandings of gender across time and place. First, we examine identities in European contexts, such as the English mollies, the Italian femminielli, Albanian sworn virgins, and multi-contextual examples of eunuchs. Such individuals were all positioned as 'other' from men and women, without necessarily being marginalised. This historical overview aims to achieve two goals—to bring the aforementioned perception of the gender binary as a 'constant' into question and, secondly, to challenge the idea that non-binary gender identities are an exclusively non-Western phenomenon.

We then consider gender on the Asian subcontinent through the Indian *hijra*, the Thai *kathoey*, and the two Indonesian examples of the *waria*, and gender within Buginese society. Finally, American examples

B. Vincent (✉) • A. Manzano
University of Leeds, Leeds, Yorkshire, UK

© The Author(s) 2017
C. Richards et al. (eds.), *Genderqueer and Non-Binary Genders*, Critical and Applied
Approaches in Sexuality, Gender and Identity, DOI 10.1057/978-1-137-51053-2_2

11

are explored with the range of two-spirit identities of First Nation tribes of the United States and Canada, and the *machi* of South America. This discussion demonstrates the heterogeneity of gender variance around the world, and how the modern Western notion of a gender binary is only one of many possible perspectives. Many of these identities are still articulated today. We conclude by briefly considering the value of cross-cultural and historical considerations beyond the gender binary. The examples selected are far from exhaustive, and geographical assumptions should not be inferred as to where gender variance may occur. For example, African (Amadiume, 1987) and Middle Eastern (Murray, 1997) examples too are well recognised.

There has been remarkable progress in the last few years regarding awareness and understanding of transgender people. Recent happenings of note include the education and activism provided by the actress Laverne Cox (Eleftheriou-Smith, 2015), together with the much discussed coming out of Caitlyn Jenner (Lutz, 2015). However, when transgender people are discussed within mainstream media, medicine, or academia, this is most often in terms of the gender binary—that is, the cultural system which positions male and female as the only possible realities. Binary transgender discourses involve the rights, experiences, and identities of people assigned male at birth that identify as women, and vice versa. Such discourses have challenged the rigidity of the gender binary, but not necessarily the possibility of being outside of it. Articulations of gender incorporating aspects of *both* male and female, neither, or alternative possibilities are, in comparison, rarely acknowledged.

The early-twentieth-century anthropological studies of non-Western cultures interpreted gendered cultural beliefs and behaviours in Western terms. The position of the Western observer-researcher was assumed as inherently 'true' and led to limited interpretations of non-Western realities (Malinowski, 1927). However, this work was of great importance in recognising cross-cultural gender variation for the first time, and one can argue that "challenging the preconception of biological sexual dimorphism" (Herdt, 1993, p. 44) was not then possible. Indeed, ethno-centric Western interpretations of gender have dominated the natural and social sciences. This background highlights the importance of discussing gender beyond contemporary Western articulations, without implying variation as 'abnormal' in relation to a Western norm. With this objective in mind, we provide a range of purposively selected cases (Blaikie, 2009) to illustrate the social construction of gender identities within European and non-Western contexts.

Global Gender Variation

Gender Transgressions, Historical Lessons: Articulations of Gender Within European Contexts

It is widely assumed that Western European societies such as the United Kingdom have always categorised people as only male and female. Genitals are assumed to be the 'essential' factor in dictating gender, and yet historically, other factors could have enough gendered significance to challenge or change an individual's status from man or woman. This relates to the important historical relationship between gender and sexuality. In the late nineteenth century, the early days of sexology, research that attempted to make sense of individuals with same-gender attraction positioned those now understood as gay men as having 'a female soul trapped in a male body' (Krafft-Ebing, 1886); however, this is now more associated with some transgender narratives. Attraction to men was viewed as so 'fundamentally female' that scientific and medical experts believed same-gender attraction challenged an individual's maleness or femaleness.

Whilst the relationship between sexuality and gender identity results in their confusion and conflation even today (Valdes, 1996), the role of sexuality in defining an individual's gender was once much more explicit. For example, Trumbach (1993) articulates how sodomy did not inherently challenge one's status as male, but being penetrated did— or similarly, if a woman penetrated other women. Thus, transgressions positioning men as submissive/penetrated or women as dominant/penetrators impacted upon gender significantly. This historical consideration also reveals how one cannot necessarily draw a clear line between binary and non-binary understandings of gender in the context of the seventeenth and eighteenth centuries. At that time, an individual's gendered status could be rendered ambiguous by factors now understood as sexual orientation, but then thought to indicate 'hermaphroditism'. 'Hermaphroditism' is an antiquated term to refer primarily to genital ambiguity, with intersex or Diversity of Sexual Development (DSD) now the term used to refer to a wide range of physiological variations.

Mollies

The term 'molly' was an eighteenth-century label associated with men attracted to other men. In addition, mollies engaged in gendered practices, which positioned them as critically separate from men who were 'othered' through their difference into a third category. Sub-cultural practices of mollies included the taking of female names and titles; marriage ceremonies between mollies; and ritualised enactments of giving birth known as 'lying-in' (Norton, 2009). Similar birthing rituals have been recognised cross-culturally—collectively referred to as *couvade* (Klein, 1991).

Eighteenth-century English society was predictably hostile towards mollies. The earlier Buggery Act of 1533 set the precedent that sodomy was punishable by death. Gaining a reputation for cross-dressing and 'sinful perversion' could result in 'social death'—whereby the individual was stigmatised and excluded from social participation. However, Norton explains how mollies' fear of stigma and execution meant "occasional 'lyings-in' could serve to relieve their collective anxiety through outrageous fun, and what today is called 'camp' behaviour" (Norton, 2009, n.p.). The behaviours of mollies served to nucleate sub-cultural associations between men who have sex with men and playfulness with gender and presentation, as contemporarily exhibited by drag queens in particular. For these reasons, one cannot simplify the molly identity or experience to that of homosexual men, or transgender women. As with any group, mollies will have been heterogeneous, with individuals differing from each other in idiosyncratic ways. Aside from this, narratives of pathology came to dominate explanations of perceived deviance in the late nineteenth and early twentieth centuries (De Block & Adriaens, 2013).

Recognising how genders were historically dependent upon orientations serves to illustrate the importance of social interaction in positioning the individual as a gendered subject. Further, the more modern categories of 'homosexual' and 'transsexual' were influenced by the older categorisations of mollies and sodomites. This illustrates the importance of recognising that "cultural context determines whether gender variation is seen as a 'disorder' needing treatment or an understood and tolerated variation" (Newman, 2002, p. 355).

Femminielli

Femminielli are specifically associated with Neapolitan culture. Zito claims that the city of Naples was historically positioned as feminine, and that connections to gendered religious rituals allowed for "Men to experience the feminine side of their nature even in a context that has always suffered the patriarchal order dating back to Greek colonisation" (Zito, 2013, p. 207). Assigned male at birth, femminielli share some gendered articulations with archetypal expectations of transgender women, such as taking a female name, and—in recent decades—accessing hormones and gender-affirming surgeries. It is only through the details of identity politics (femminielli who specifically disidentify with the notion of being transgender women) and specific cultural practices that differentiation can be seen. For example, Atlas describes how femminielli could articulate themselves in specific ways, which would be frowned upon if done by women or men in Naples:

> Normally men are not allowed at the *tombola* because trousers worn at the game (i.e. the presence of men) would bring bad luck. Lella [a femminielli] disagreed, arguing that transvestites like her, who wore trousers, were allowed in. (Atlas, 2005, p. 55)

Whilst women would not wear trousers, and men would not be allowed to attend the *tombola* (a bingo-like game), the specific way in which femminielli are culturally integrated and involved allows for femminielli to occupy a third gender position. In a similar way to Lella herself in the above quotation, some scholars argue that the femminielli no longer truly exist today, but may be understood as transvestites (D'Amora, 2013). However, this risks erasing the specific context within which the category of femminielli was negotiated over time, as well as those femminielli who do not identify with the labels of transvestite or transgender. This demonstrates the fluidity of gender, as individuals may have overlapping or seemingly contradictory identifications—some femminielli identifying themselves as men who dress as women, whilst others identify as neither men nor women.

Another important difference from binary transgender narratives is the complex relationship with stigma. Whilst traditional Neapolitan culture polices gender roles, femminielli are not disciplined for breach of these cultural rules due to their specific social position. Indeed, whilst many contemporary transgender and non-binary narratives indicate experiences of discrimination, abuse, and rejection, femminielli are often accepted within communities, sometimes living with their immediate or extended family. Femminielli are also believed to bring luck, due to historical association with the deity Hermaphroditus (Piraino & Zambelli, 2015). Therefore, specific details of the Neapolitan context directly influenced the development of the femminielli as an expression of gender variance.

Sworn Virgins

In Albanian tribes, having a son to continue the family line was of great cultural, social, and financial importance, not least because only males were eligible to inherit property. Families lacking a son would lose their property as their family name became extinct. However, they could resist and avoid this through the social construction of a son, from a child assigned female at birth. This occurred either at birth (in the case of single-child families) or in cases where an older son was lost: "the biological female who, later in life, after having been socialized as a woman for many years, reconstructs herself as a 'social man'" (Grémaux, 1993, p. 244). Today, the practice of sworn virginity is near extinction. Whilst limited research makes estimation difficult, as few as some dozen sworn virgins may still live after Albanian communism prevented the continuation of many traditional practices (Becatoros, 2008). Cultural shifts over the twentieth century and the relaxation of patriarchal limitations on women's rights have also diminished the social relevance of sworn virginity. Whilst the legitimacy of sworn virgins as male was seen through their inclusion in male-only social spaces and practices, communities did perceive a difference from other men. Grémaux's ethnographic research involved talking to Albanian elders who knew the sworn virgin Mikas, who died in 1934. In discussing Mikas, "informants alternately used 'he' and 'she', as was observed by Gusic [an earlier ethnographer] when Mikas was still alive" (Grémaux, 1993, p. 251).

The issue of virginity itself was surprisingly flexible, depending upon ethno-social group membership. Marriage was the consistent taboo, due to creating an unacceptable male/male partnership. That Albanian sworn virgins could discuss attraction to women in male social circles emphasises the social validity/reality of the assumed third gender category, whilst simultaneously reifying culturally dominant heteronormativity and patriarchy. Thus, the nuances of social acceptability and gendered difference as a legitimised expression of gender variation were highly dependent on idiosyncratic considerations of gender and sexuality in that context.

Eunuchs

Commonly referring to castrated men, eunuchs were found in a range of different cultures serving different specific functions. In the Ottoman Empire, for example, many male slaves were eunuchs; however, within Chinese and Roman contexts, eunuchs could act as powerful civil servants (Tsai, 1996). Eunuchs were seen as less likely to attempt to overthrow reigning leadership due to their inability to have children and continue a lineage.

Ringrose explains how within Byzantine society the definition of eunuch changed over time, originally referring to "anyone who did not, as well as could not, produce children, including men who were born sterile, men who became sterile through illness, accident or birth defect, men who were lacking in sexual desire and men and women who embraced the celibate life for religious reasons" (Ringrose, 1993). Thus, 'eunuch' within this historical context had a much broader meaning than is now generally appreciated. In some circumstances, castration was chosen and

desired. Such individuals included priests for ritual purposes or to inter-
act with women more freely, or scholars who believed the loss of 'vital
fluids' through ejaculation might hamper the intellect. The form of castration could also differ, with some experiencing *total ablation*—removal
of the penis and testes to prevent sexual relations with court ladies they
were to protect and/or serve. For example, removal of the penis was common in China, but not in Rome (Scheidel, 2009).

It is debatable whether eunuchs were considered men or not, and
indeed this may have always been a grey area in some of those historical
contexts. Castration did, however, function to transform the individual
into one distinctly 'other' (and often less) than 'whole' men, in order to
perform socially constructed functions for which men and women were
deemed unsuitable. Whilst historical records show much negative senti-
ment directed towards eunuchs, particularly lacking in strength, bravery,
and stoicism associated with whole men, they could arrive at social positions of acceptance or even power. In the Byzantine Empire, eunuchs
could often be well educated, with various court positions reserved specifically for them. Eunuchs could be favoured in some cultures as performers. Indeed, the castration of boys to maintain their high vocal registers
in Catholic choirs was only made illegal in Italy in 1870. The example
of eunuchs highlights how maleness has been tied to masculinity, which
has been constructed through a range of factors. Some of these have had
cross-cultural significance such as fertility and physical stature, though
the importance of any given factor may be idiosyncratic.

This section has demonstrated that there has been a wide range of systems for considering gender historically within European societies. Whilst
some of these experienced stigma and discrimination, it is important to
recognise how gender variation could sometimes also be constructed as a
'normal' difference within particular settings.

Around the World in 80 Genders: Examples of Gender Diversity in Non-Western Civilisations

As cultural contexts shift and evolve, so do gendered possibilities. This is
evidenced when considering non-Western gender variances. This section

is structured geographically, beginning with considerations of gender across Asia before moving to the Americas. Unlike most of the European examples, all of the cases discussed in this section may still be found within their respective societies today, although—predictably—differences in their articulations have occurred over time. It is also worth considering how these non-Western identities have been affected by modern Western influences, with colonialism of particular salience to the Indian and North American discussions. We begin with the *hijra* who, whilst the term may be literally translated as 'eunuch' (or sometimes 'hermaphrodite') differ greatly from the European discussion.

Hijra

The *hijra* illustrate a gender identity that is situated in relation to both the caste system and the practice of Hinduism across the Indian subcontinent. Thus, the *hijra* exemplify how intersections between class, culture, faith, and other factors can shape different identity categories. *Hijra* can be subcategorised—with *born hijra* typically possessing ambiguous genitalia at birth (as with some—though not all—intersex individuals), and *made hijra* who often come to their identity in part through a lack of attraction to women—historically positioning them as 'incomplete men'. This delineation is by no means sufficient, as *hijra* also disidentify both with being male and masculinity. *Hijra* community structure is based around communes, which are part of larger city networks. Households will have leaders or *gurus* who function to organise the finances collected from the work of the *hijra* within the house, and prospective *hijra* require sponsorship from a guru (Nanda, 1993). Many *hijra* undergo an operation (traditionally by another *hijra*) to remove the penis and testicles, without vaginal construction. This defines the *hijra* as neither man nor woman (Nanda, 1990).

The origin of the *hijra* and their practice of castration are strongly associated with Hindu beliefs and practices. The *hijra* community is centred around the worship of Bahuchara Mata, a *mother goddess* deity. The practice of castration and feminine identification originated with the story of the goddess appearing in a dream to an impotent prince and ordering him to remove his genitals and serve her as a woman or experience divine punishment. It is through the Hindu faith that the *hijra* were able to gain cultural legitimacy as ritual performers for important events (such as births, festivals, and weddings). Whilst this legitimacy translated into recent recognition under Indian law through creation of a third gender category on Indian passports, *hijra* can simultaneously be heavily stigmatised. This is, in part, due to the incorporation of norms related to gender and sexual orientation through British colonialism. The British removed state protection from the *hijra*, described their roles as "abominable practices of the wretches", and passed "laws criminalizing emasculation" which would remain after Indian independence (Nanda, 1993, p. 414).

More recently, ritual practices in India have become shorter and increasingly nonessential and as a result, *hijra* communities have relied increasingly upon organised begging and sex work (Chakrapani, Babu, & Ebenezer, 2004). Those *hijra* households who engage in sex work will utilise the guru in an analogous manner to a pimp or madam, which may allow for a significant rise in household income. There is also a sense that such practices are offensive to the traditional *hijra* role, and *hijra* may have their living quarters separated based on who does and who does not engage in sex work, indicating how *hijra* identity and meaning are changing over time (Wilson, 2006).

Kathoey

The term *kathoey* is used to refer to individuals assigned male at birth, but can have diverse meanings. For some, *kathoey* are analogous with effeminate gay men, whilst for others, similar to transgender women. Many *kathoey* identify simply as female (*phuying*), whilst others as "a second kind of female" (*phuying prophet song*), others yet simply as *kathoey*, articulated as a third category separate from male and female (Winter, 2006). One commonality seems to be that *kathoey* individuals think of themselves as "something other than male". Some *kathoey* access oestrogen and surgeries (such as breast implants and facial feminisation) whilst embracing a highly feminine style. Others may mix category-associated expectations, such as by wearing 'male clothes' together with makeup, and using female pronouns.

Käng (2012) explains how the Thai state formalised legal restrictions on gendered presentation and dress, due to Western views of Thai women as transgressively androgynous. *Kathoey* may sometimes be translated into English as the term 'ladyboy', which within a Thai context can imply association with particular economies, such as cabaret or sex work. Whilst some *kathoey* use ladyboy without issue, others may be offended—as the word can be taken to imply that they are sex workers (Käng, 2012). However, some *kathoey* certainly do engage in sex work, corresponding with Harrison, Grant and Herman's (2012) study evidencing that Western non-binary identified people are more likely than the general population to be involved in 'underground economies', including sex work. Consideration of HIV risk and drug use amongst *kathoey* individuals illustrates the vulnerability of the group (Nemoto et al., 2012). This can be linked to stigmatisation within Thai society, resulting in potential family rejection and difficulty accessing legal forms of work.

Ten Brummelhuis stated that "Most *kathoey* I interviewed estimated that about twenty-five percent of their [male] partners are not aware they are transgender males [*sic*]" (1999, p. 129). This linguistic positioning of *kathoey* as male rests upon a biological essentialism which obscures both how they are viewed by others and themselves. This illustrates the importance of accommodating a culturally specific understanding of gender variance into clinical and social research aiming to access and assist vulnerable members of a society.

Waria and the Buginese People

Waria possess many comparable traits with the *kathoey*. The label is derived from combining the words *wanita* or woman, and *pria*, or man (Boellstorff, 2004), and can refer to a range of articulations of feminine identity and practice amongst individuals assigned male at birth. The different ethno-social groups found amongst the island nation of Indonesia means that the origins of *waria* are uncertain. There are accounts from the 1820s of "transvestite performers" (Boellstorff, 2004, p. 164), and by the 1960s, *waria* were well known, through association with sex work. Boellstorff explains how *waria* can be differentiated from Western notions of cross-dressers and transgender women:

> To only be interested in women's clothes or activities is not usually seen as sufficient to make one waria; at some point, usually while a child but sometimes in the teenage years, waria come to know that they have the soul (*jiwa*) of a woman, or at least a soul that is more woman than man … the goal is not to 'pass' but to look like a waria. (Boellstorff, 2004, p. 167)

Whilst surgery is rarely desired, hormones and other practices (such as skin whitening creams) are used, which allows agency over the construction of gender presentation. Such practices can be associated with structural racism (the status whiteness holds in relation to beauty) and harm from chemical use (Idrus & Hymans, 2014).

In contrast to *waria*, who can be related in part to Western transgender narratives, the Buginese people (an ethnic group found on the island of Sulawesi, Indonesia's third largest) have a social system accommodating five gender categories. Whilst a detailed analysis of spiritual practices, specific gender roles, historical context, dress, and interactions would be necessary for a full explanation, it can be noted that some of these categories are analogous with Western conceptualisations. Two of the five genders of the Buginese are the oroané and makkunrai which are analogous to cisgender[1] men and women, respectively. The further three genders include the calabai, who are individuals assigned male at birth but who live as heterosexual women, whilst the calalai are assigned female at birth but live as heterosexual men. There is (perhaps predictably) slippage in the precision of such definitions, illustrated by one calabai who said "some calabai like women, but they're not real calabai" (Graham, 2004, p. 113). Finally, there are the bissu, who are considered a combination of man and woman within an empowering cultural-spiritual narrative. The *waria* and the Buginese illuminate how different non-binary gender systems can simultaneously be articulated within a single nation.

Two-Spirit People

'Two-spirit' is a relatively recent umbrella term used to refer to a range of roles and identities amongst different indigenous North Americans—including the Winkte of the Lakota, the Nàdleehi of the Navajo, and the Badés of the Sioux amongst others. The term replaces the word 'berdache', which was used in earlier literature. 'Berdache' had its origins in the French for 'male prostitute' and is now considered an inappropriate slur—a cultural sensitivity which anthropological researchers did not historically consider (Epple, 1998).

In the past, rituals which assigned two-spirit people their gender status allowed for those individuals to engage with forms of dress, social activities, and labour usually reserved for those tribes-folk of the 'opposite' physiological category to that of the two-spirit person. The binarised nature of language when discussing gender in English makes it difficult to do justice to non-Western social systems, which have culturally embedded articulations of gender beyond the binary. Simplifications and concessions must occasionally be made, but it is important to recognise that whilst in a Western context a two-spirit person with a penis may have been assigned male at birth, it is problematic to apply this framework of understanding to Native American infants when processes of socialisation (particularly historically) were different. For example, the North American Zuni tribe did not position an immediate view of physiology as the primary indicator of gender. Ritual interventions during pregnancy and after the birth were understood as essential for the development of gender. Roscoe describes how:

> The midwife massaged and manipulated the infant's face, nose, eyes and genitals. If the infant was male, she poured cold water over its penis to prevent overdevelopment. If the child was female, the midwife split a new gourd in half and rubbed it over the vulva to enlarge it. In this context, knowing the kind of genitals an individual possesses is less important than knowing how bodies are culturally constructed and what particular features and processes (physiological and/or social) are believed to endow them with sex. (Roscoe, 1993, pp. 342–343)

Some tribes might understand the individual to possess two identities articulated at different times, thus the origin of the name 'two-spirit'. This allowed for 'men's clothing' to be worn on some occasions and 'women's clothing' on others. Two-spirit people would occupy positions of social respect (though how this was articulated was tribally dependent), and were often thought to have spiritual powers.

Not all tribes regarded their two-spirited members with universal respect, as association with supernatural practices could render some two-spirit people subjects of fear. Occupying positions of respect also did not render two-spirit people as beyond criticism or punishment (Walker, 1982); however, the roles of third genders in Native American tribes were integral, typical, and substantial.

Machi

The *machi* are found within the Mapuche indigenous group, located across parts of Chile and Argentina. Similar to the *hijra* and some two-spirit people, *machi* have religious significance within their communities, and are positioned as shamans with healing powers. Their gender variance is strongly tied to ritualism, with Bacigalupo explaining the sacred use of the Foye tree, and how "Its white, hermaphroditic flowers legitimate *machi's* ritual transvestism, their sexual variance, and their co-gendered ritual identities (during rituals they move between masculine and feminine gender polarities or combine the two)" (Bacigalupo, 2010).

In contrast to earlier examples, *machi* identity construction is strongly context specific and changeable. This fluidity is also manifest in insider/outsider dynamics with regards to Mapuche identity, involving complex interactions between race, language, ancestry, knowledge, and colonial influences (Bacigalupo, 2003). The articulations of gender variance amongst the *machi* have also been constrained through interactions with westernised, non-Mapuche Chilean society. Fine-Dare (2014) positions this constraint as a duality between expression of a gendered fluidity, whilst also needing to defend and resist masculinity and femininity in binarised terms in particular interactions, such as providing healing services for outsiders. Bacigalupo illustrates how expression of stigmatised gender variance in non-Mapuche Chilean society is policed by recounting how one *machi* who was read as male but identified as female was "jailed without trial under a false accusation of homicide. Additionally she was described as a 'strange sexual deviant' and a 'dangerous uncivilized Indian' because she challenged Chilean gender and social norms"

(Bacigalupo, 2003, p. 37). Whilst stigma and discrimination based on gender identity and race are still tragically common within Western contexts, the way in which gender, race, and nationality intersect within the context of the Mapuche must be considered specifically in order to appreciate the nuances of the local social geography.

Conclusion

Throughout this chapter, we have attempted to demonstrate how fluid, fuzzy, and ultimately difficult to categorise diverse articulations of gender can be, when thinking in terms of the gender binary. Indeed, whilst stigma and discrimination can drive gender and sexuality minorities underground, there is no reason to believe such articulations cannot be found in any and all nations and contexts. Themes can be observed across articulations of gender variance such as being regarded as lucky, sacred, as leaders, or (and sometimes simultaneously) how gender variance can increase the likelihood of experiencing stigmatisation or risk—particularly in relation to sex work.

The benefits of considering gender diversity lie in appreciating how particular contexts can result in highly varied articulations of gender. This can be harnessed so as to lessen gendered assumptions within service provision. This is particularly important given that gender variant people are more likely to experience economic and social vulnerability, and may struggle to have health needs taken seriously, or addressed appropriately. Further, gender variant people are not necessary visibly identifiable.

By increasing awareness of gender variance, greater specificity may be attained when assisting those who present themselves as defying normative gender expectations. Conversations about binary transgender issues are vitally important, and there remains much work still to be done in combating stigma and discrimination. However, whilst there is huge variation in how transgender people who identify within the gender binary articulate themselves (i.e. as men and women), this is only one facet of the remarkable breadth of gendered possibility, both inside and beyond Western cultural contexts.

Summary

* The idea that gender is only experienced individually and culturally as 'man or woman' is a relatively recent, Western idea.
* 'Biological' and 'cultural' aspects of gender cannot be disentangled, and attempts to do so risk essentialising particular factors above others and delegitimising some experiences of gender variance.
* Explanations of gender variance in terms of the gender binary can result in the loss of specific details dependent on their cultural context.
* Gender variance and sexuality are now conceived separately in a Western context, but historically and cross-culturally they have been entwined.
* Many cultures understand gender in terms differing from the gender binary. These identities can illustrate how gender variance may be celebrated, but patterns of social vulnerability and stigma are present.

Notes

1. *Cisgender* refers to men and women who identify with the gender they were assigned at birth. The term has gained prominence as it challenges the assumption that the words *men* and *women* implicitly exclude trans people, and avoids positioning cisgender status as 'normal', and transgender by implication as 'abnormal'.

References

Amadiume, I. (1987). *Male Daughters, Female Husbands: Gender and Sex in an African Society*. London: Zed Books.

Atlas, M. (2005). Representing Femminelli of Naples. *FKW//Zeitschrift für Geschlechterforschung und visuelle Kultur, 37*(39), 52–58.

Bacigalupo, A. M. (2003). Rethinking Identity and Feminism: Contributions of Mapuche Women and Machi from Southern Chile. *Hypatia, 18*(2), 32–57.

Bacigalupo, A. M. (2010). *Shamans of the Foye Tree: Gender, Power, and Healing Among Chilean Mapuche*. Austin: University of Texas Press.

Becatoros, E. (2008). *Tradition of 'Sworn Virgins' Dying Out in Albania*. Retrieved June 21, 2015, from http://www.welt.de/english-news/article2536539/Tradition-of-sworn-virgins-dying-out-in-Albania.html

Blaikie, N. (2009). *Designing Social Research* (2nd ed.). Cambridge: Polity Press.

Boellstorff, T. (2004). Playing Back the Nation: Waria, Indonesian Transvestites. *Cultural Anthropology, 19*(2), 159–195.

Chakrapani, V., Babu, P., & Ebenezer, T. (2004). Hijras in Sex Work Face Discrimination in the Indian Health-Care System. *Research for Sex Work, 7*, 12–14.

D'Amora, M. (2013). La figura del femminiello/travestito nella cultura e nel teatro contemporaneo napoletano. *Cahiers d'études italiennes, 16*, 201–212.

De Block, A., & Adriaens, P. R. (2013). Pathologizing Sexual Deviance: A History. *Journal of Sex Research, 50*(3–4), 276–298.

Eleftheriou-Smith, L.-M. (2015). *Laverne Cox Says Focus on Transgender People Needs to Shift From Before-and-After of Surgery: 'It Objectifies Us, Reducing Us to Our Bodies'*. Retrieved July 18, 2015, from http://www.independent.co.uk/news/people/laverne-cox-says-focus-on-transgender-people-needs-to-shift-from-beforeandafter-of-surgery-it-objectifies-us-reducing-us-to-our-bodies-10387689.html

Epple, C. (1998). Coming to Terms with Navajo Nádleehí: A Critique of Berdache, "Gay," "Alternate Gender," and "Two Spirit". *American Ethnologist, 25*(2), 267–290.

Fine-Dare, K. (2014). Ritualized Dimensions of Personhood, Sociality, and Power Among the Mapuche of Chile. *Latin American and Caribbean Ethnic Studies, 9*(3), 356–361.

Graham, S. (2004). It's Like One of Those Puzzles: Conceptualising Gender Among Bugis. *Journal of Gender Studies, 13*(2), 107–116.

Grémaux, R. (1993). Woman Becomes Man in the Balkans. In G. Herdt (Ed.), *Third Sex, Third Gender: Beyond Sexual Dimorphism in Culture and History*. New York: Zone Books.

Harrison, J., Grant, J., & Herman, J. L. (2012). A Gender Not Listed Here: Genderqueers, Gender Rebels, and Otherwise in the National Transgender Discrimination Survey. *LGBTQ Public Policy Journal at the Harvard Kennedy School, 2*(1), 13–24.

Herdt, G. H. (1993). *Third Sex, Third Gender: Beyond Sexual Dimorphism in Culture and History*. New York: Zone Books.

Idrus, N. I., & Hymans, T. D. (2014). Balancing Benefits and Harm: Chemical Use and Bodily Transformation Among Indonesia's Transgender Waria. *The International Journal on Drug Policy, 25*(4), 789–797.

Käng, D. B. C. (2012). Kathoey "In Trend": Emergent Genderscapes, National Anxieties and the Re-Signification of Male-Bodied Effeminacy in Thailand. *Asian Studies Review, 36*(4), 475–494.

Klein, H. (1991). Couvade Syndrome: Male Counterpart to Pregnancy. *The International Journal of Psychiatry in Medicine, 21*(1), 57–69.

Krafft-Ebing, R. V. (1886). *Psychopathia Sexualis* (F. S. Klaf, Trans.). New York: Arcade Publishing.

Lutz, T. (2015). *Caitlyn Jenner Accepts Courage Award: 'If You Want to Call Me Names, I Can Take It'*. Retrieved July 18, 2015, from http://www.theguardian.com/sport/2015/jul/15/caitlyn-jenner-receives-espy-award-and-says-transgender-people-deserve-respect

Malinowski, B. (1927). *Sex and Repression in Savage Society*. London: Kegan Paul, Trench, Trubner & Co.

Murray, S. O. (1997). The Sohari Khanith. In S. O. Murray & W. Roscoe (Eds.), *Islamic Homosexualities: Culture, History, and Literature* (pp. 256–261). New York: New York University Press.

Nanda, S. (1990). *Neither Man Nor Woman: The Hijras of India*. Belmont, CA: Wadsworth Publishing.

Nanda, S. (1993). Hijras: An Alternative Sex and Gender Role in India. In G. Herdt (Ed.), *Third Sex Third Gender: Beyond Sexual Dimorphism in Culture and History* (pp. 373–418). New York: Zone Books.

Nemoto, T., Iwamoto, M., Perngparn, U., Areesantichai, C., Kamitani, E., & Sakata, M. (2012). HIV-Related Risk Behaviors Among Kathoey (Male-to-Female Transgender) Sex Workers in Bangkok, Thailand. *AIDS Care, 24*(2), 210–219.

Newman, L. K. (2002). Sex, Gender and Culture: Issues in the Definition, Assessment and Treatment of Gender Identity Disorder. *Clinical Child Psychology and Psychiatry, 7*(3), 352–359.

Norton, R. (2009). *Maiden Names and Little Sports*. The Gay Subculture in Georgian England. Retrieved June 20, 2015, from http://rictornorton.co.uk/eighteen/maiden.htm

Piraino, F., & Zambelli, L. (2015). Santa Rosalia and Mamma Schiavona: Popular Worship Between Religiosity and Identity. *Critical Research on Religion*. doi:10.1177/2050303215593150.

Ringrose, K. M. (1993). Living in the Shadows: Eunuchs and Gender in Byzantium. In G. Herdt (Ed.), *Third Sex Third Gender: Beyond Sexual Dimorphism in Culture and History*. New York: Zone Books.

Roscoe, W. (1993). How to Become a Berdache: Toward a Unified Analysis of Gender Diversity. In G. Herdt (Ed.), *Third Sex, Third Gender: Beyond Sexual Dimorphism in Culture and History*. New York: Zone Books.

Scheidel, W. (Ed.). (2009). *Rome and China: Comparative Perspectives on Ancient World Empires*. Oxford: Oxford University Press.

Ten Brummelhuis, H. (1999). Transformations of Transgender: The Case of the Thai Kathoey. *Journal of Gay & Lesbian Social Services, 9*(2–3), 121–139.

Trumbach, R. (1993). London's Sapphists: From Three Sexes to Four Genders in the Making of Modern Culture. In G. Herdt (Ed.), *Third Sex Third Gender: Beyond Sexual Dimorphism in Culture and History*. New York: Zone Books.

Tsai, S. S. H. (1996). *The Eunuchs in the Ming Dynasty*. Albany: State University of New York Press.

Valdes, F. (1996). Unpacking Hetero-Patriarchy: Tracing the Conflation of Sex, Gender & Sexual Orientation to Its Origins. *Yale Journal of Law and the Humanities, 8*, 161–212.

Walker, J. R. (1982). *Lakota Society*. Lincoln: University of Nebraska Press.

Wilson, N. A. (2006). The Modernization of Hijras. *Journal of Scholarship and Opinion, 6*, 33–40.

Winter, S. (2006). Thai Transgenders in Focus: Demographics, Transitions and Identities. *International Journal of Transgenderism, 9*(1), 15–27.

Zito, E. (2013). Disciplinary Crossings and Methodological Contaminations in Gender Research: A Psycho-Anthropological Survey on Neapolitan Femminielli. *International Journal of Multiple Research Approaches, 7*(2), 204–217.

Further Reading

Herdt, G. H. (1993). *Third Sex, Third Gender: Beyond Sexual Dimorphism in Culture and History*. New York: Zone Books.

Johnston, L. (2015). Gender and Sexuality I Genderqueer Geographies? *Progress in Human Geography*, 1–11.

Kessler, S. J. & McKenna, W. (1978). *Gender: An Ethnomethodological Approach* (Chap. 2). In *Cross-Cultural Perspectives on Gender* (pp. 21–42). Chicago: University of Chicago Press.

Newman, L. K. (2002). Sex, Gender and Culture: Issues in the Definition, Assessment and Treatment of Gender Identity Disorder. *Clinical Child Psychology and Psychiatry*, *7*, 352–359.

Ochoa, M. (2008). Perverse Citizenship: Divas, Marginality, and Participation in "Loca-Lization". *WSQ: Women's Studies Quarterly*, *36*, 146–169.

3

Non-binary Activism

S. Bear Bergman and Meg-John Barker

Introduction

This chapter introduces the burgeoning non-binary gender movement. Meg-John Barker writes the first half of the chapter, which is a summary of non-binary activism with a particular focus on the UK as an illustrative example of the kind of work that is happening in this area. Meg-John begins by charting some of the history of the non-binary movement and overviews the areas which have been focal points for activism so far. They also set out some of the main forms of activism which are currently taking place in the UK context and look to what the future might hold. Meg-John then passes over to Canada-based trans activist S. Bear

S. Bear Bergman
Toronto, Canada

M.-J. Barker (✉)
The Open University, Milton Keynes, Buckinghamshire, UK

© The Author(s) 2017
C. Richards et al. (eds.), *Genderqueer and Non-Binary Genders*, Critical and Applied
Approaches in Sexuality, Gender and Identity, DOI 10.1057/978-1-137-51053-2_3

Bergman who is more familiar with the US and Canadian context. Bear provides a personal reflection on experiences of activism around non-binary identity, in relation to language in particular. This is an important area of focus given the binary gendered nature of the English language (and many others), and the commonality of linguistic misgendering and microaggressions in the everyday lives of many non-binary people.

Overview of Non-binary Activism So Far

Meg-John Barker

A New Movement?

In the period when we were writing this chapter in early 2016, two events happened in the UK which raised important questions about how new the non-binary movement is: Kate Bornstein's series of public talks and performances across UK cities in February (Saner, 2016) and the combined non-binary conference and trans studies SexGen North seminar at Leeds University in March (Hines, 2016; Vincent & Erikainen, 2016).

The non-binary gender movement is frequently hailed as a new phenomenon, with people pointing particularly to the Facebook gender 'revolution' in 2014 as a starting point of public attention (Richards, 2014). Certainly, Google's Ngram viewer, which graphically represents the frequency of mentions of words or phrases in published texts, provides no results for *non-binary gender* prior to its current endpoint of 2008, whilst *transgender* sees a huge climb from nowhere the late 1980s to 2008, and *genderqueer* a small increase from nothing in the mid 2000s.

However, key figures in trans activism since the very earliest days of that movement, Kate Bornstein and Stephen Whittle, both made very similar points at the 2016 events: that trans activism had been challenging the gender binary right from the start, and that they certainly hadn't experienced their own genders in purely binary ways (see Bornstein, 1994; Whittle, 1996). This perhaps explains why, although not always entirely comfortable, the reception of non-binary activism by broader trans activism has so far been a good deal more welcoming than the historical reception of bisexual activism by broader gay/LGB rights movements (see Barker, Richards, Jones, Bowes-Catton, & Plowman, 2012).

The discussion which followed at these events encouraged us to hold various paradoxes and tensions in relation to the non-binary moment. We need to understand its place as a very new social movement which, like the asexual movement (Carrigan, Gupta, & Morrison, 2013), has only reached critical mass in recent times due to the potentials afforded by the internet for collective engagement across geographical location. At the same time, we need to trace non-binary activism back through time via the trans, queer, and bisexual movements which have been challenging binaries of sex, gender, and sexuality for some decades now (e.g. see Bornstein & Bergman, 2010; Nestle & Wilchins, 2002; Queen & Schimel, 1997) and through earlier forms of feminism which did similar things (e.g. see Bem & Lewis, 1975; Piercy, 1976). Similarly, it's important to chart the longer histories of non-binary gender experience which have often been erased through the centuries (Gust, 2016) in order to legitimise the movement and to provide some sense of liveable non-binary lives. However, it is also important to recognise the risks that doing so may involve reading the present onto the past in problematic ways analogous with viewing culturally diverse gender experiences through the colonising lens of Western understanding (see Vincent & Manzano-Santaella, this volume).

Areas of Focus

Thus far, the following areas seem to have formed focal points for non-binary activism. I've provided UK references to exemplify each of these, which I will go on to discuss further in the next section (note that I've dated these as if they are an ongoing website or blog, but many began before the dates given here).

* Conducting and reporting grass-roots research with non-binary people to obtain statistics regarding the prevalence of non-binary people and the challenges they face, in order that activism can be grounded in persuasive evidence (e.g. Barker & Lester, 2015; Breaking the Binary, 2016; Titman, 2014; Valentine, 2016)

- Campaigning for the rights of non-binary people to self-determine their gender and to have their gender accurately recorded in documentation which displays gender, such as passports and organisational records, or to have gender markers removed entirely from such documentation (e.g. Elan-Cane, 2015; Non-binary Inclusion Project, 2016; Stonewall, 2015; see also Clucus & Whittle, this volume)
- Activism around language to ensure that, for example, the gender neutral title 'Mx' is provided as an option by banks and other institutions, and that social and mainstream media include gender neutral pronouns such as 'they,' and recognise these as legitimate (see Bennet, 2016; Tobia, 2015)
- Awareness-raising and education to improve cultural understanding, and media coverage, of non-binary people (e.g. All About Trans, 2016; Trans Media Watch, 2014), and to encourage better support of those whose gender intersects with other marginalised identities (e.g. Choudrey, 2016)
- Providing support and resources for non-binary people themselves (e.g. Beyond the Binary, 2016; Breaking the binaries, 2016; Gendered Intelligence, 2013; Genderqueer in the UK, 2016; Howitt, 2016; Lester, 2015; Non-binary Scotland, 2016; nonbinary.org, 2016a)
- Working towards non-binary people being provided with easy access to National Health Service (NHS) medical services through general practitioners and gender identity clinics, and helping those who are currently struggling to access such services (e.g. Action for Trans Health, 2016; Large, 2016; Lorimer, 2016; Non-binary Inclusion Project, 2016; see also elsewhere in this volume)
- Attempts to make public spaces such as toilets and changing rooms gender neutral or non-binary inclusive (see Cambridge University Students' Union LGBT+ Campaign, 2016; Sanghani, 2015)
- Provision of non-binary specific, and non-binary inclusive, social and supportive spaces (e.g. Be: Non-Binary, 2016; Non-binary London, 2016; Open Barbers, 2016; Wotever World, 2016)
- Inclusion of non-binary people in wider trans activist campaigns around topics such as prisons (see Lees, 2016), hate crime (see Galop, 2011), and asylum seeking (see UKLGIG, 2016)

UK Non-binary Activism So Far

It's important to point out that one exciting feature of non-binary activism is the tendency to challenge and blur other binaries beyond just the gender binary. For example, the *Moving Beyond the Binaries* conference (Vincent & Erikainen, 2016) was an explicitly activist-academic event (Barker, 2015) including many speakers who occupied multiple positions as activists, academics, and artists, and spoke about these intersecting roles in their presentations (e.g. Lester, 2016; White, 2016). Many non-binary activists also weave together their personal stories with their activist campaigning in innovative ways, and this is important in providing those who access their blogs, videos, podcasts, music, and artwork with visible models of what a liveable non-binary life might look like (e.g. Howitt, 2016; Lester, 2015). Increasing numbers of therapists, medics, psychologists, and psychiatrists are open about their own non-binary identities and/or are working directly towards better services for non-binary people (e.g. Lorimer, 2016, and the practitioners included within this volume). Indeed, I asked on the UK Pink Therapy Facebook network last year whether any other non-binary therapists would be interested in forming a supportive group, and this group is already at 13 members.

There have been many key moments in UK non-binary activism in recent years, where non-binary voices have explicitly been included in wider debates and trans campaigning. Here is just a brief selection of these:

In 2014, the then LGB charity Stonewall conducted a trans consultation prior to becoming trans-inclusive, and non-binary people were one of the groups who were specifically consulted with a separate non-binary specific event (Stonewall, 2015). They now include non-binary-identified staff within their organisation.

In July 2015, Ashley Reed launched a 30,000 signatory online petition asking the UK to join the growing list of countries (Ireland, Italy, Argentina, etc.) which allow trans people to self-define their gender rather than having to pay to go through a Gender Recognition Panel. The petition was inclusive of non-binary people. The Ministry of Justice responded that it would not open up certification to non-binary people because only "a very small number of people consider themselves to be of neither gender" and "we are not aware that that results in any specific detriment." Thus, the twitter hashtag #specificdetriment was born out of non-binary people contesting this response, and two large surveys were quickly conducted to provide evidence regarding the prevalence of non-binary gender and the specific detriments experienced by non-binary people (Beyond the Binary, 2015; ScottishTrans.org, 2016). CN Lester and I were asked by a group of trans activists to attend a meeting with the Ministry of Justice, where we presented the initial qualitative *Beyond the Binary* findings along with previous data regarding the relatively high levels of mental health difficulties among non-binary people (Barker & Lester, 2015). Valentine (2016) has since analysed the largescale quantitative study that ScottishTrans.org conducted which found that, for example, over three quarters of non-binary people avoid situations for fear of being misgendered, outed, or harassed; and two thirds feel that they are never included in services, with very few feel able to be out at work.

In January 2016, the UK House of Commons Women and Equalities Commission published the Trans Equality Report, which was the result of a long inquiry that included evidence from many non-binary individuals, activists, and experts. The report called for more extensive investigation into the needs of non-binary people; for a gender X option to be added to passports (in addition to M and F) and to move away from gender markers on passports long-term; for non-binary people to be protected from discrimination under the gender Equality Act; and for updating of trans medical procedures to be inclusive of non-binary people (see also NHS England, 2015).

Of course, this is just the tip of the iceberg of UK non-binary activism given that much of it occurs behind the scenes of such public engagements: in social media networks; in quick responses to relevant media representations or smaller policy decisions; and in bottom-up work that happens in classrooms, workplaces, LGBT+ centres, and other communities and institutions across the country. Recent examples that I'm personally aware of include calls for the Memorandum of Understanding of UK therapy organisations against conversion therapy to be inclusive of trans and non-binary people; and engagement with a series of proposed national and international non-binary-related programming in an attempt to shift the narrative from debates over the existence of non-binary people to a focus on diverse non-binary experiences with no requirement of a "counter-point" position from somebody who is sceptical about non-binary gender. In Wales, a group of young people, including non-binary teens, have co-produced an illustrated guide on how young people can creatively and safely campaign for gender equity and diversity. As part of this, they included The Rotifer Project, in which a Gender Play teacher workshop and assembly was designed by young people to demonstrate the diversity of gender and how damaging it can be to box people into gender categories that don't fit. They created various playful activities including GenderSnap cards with examples of gender diverse creatures, characters, and historical figures.[1]

Where Do We Go from Here?

Regarding the future, it was clear from discussions at the Leeds conference and seminar (Hines, 2016; Vincent & Erikainen, 2016) that it is vital to campaign across many of the existing strands of activism simultaneously. Both Valentine (2016) and Whittle (2016) stressed the remaining dangers inherent in endeavouring to openly occupy a non-binary gender (in terms of expression and identity), and the particular risk for those whose gender intersects with other marginalised identities and experiences (more feminine-presenting, BAME, disabled, intersex, and working class non-binary people, for example). Therefore, any moves towards legal recognition of non-binary gender need to be combined with increased education and cultural awareness, and protection from discrimination and harassment for non-binary people.

From the outside, the non-binary movement is often regarded as both 'young' and 'difficult.' Discussion of non-binary gender has often occurred within considerations of controversial social justice campaigning tactics such as 'no-platforming,' insistence on provision of 'trigger warnings,' and 'call-out culture.' These, in addition to campaigns around changing language, are often presented as threats to "freedom of speech" and as 'political correctness gone mad' (see Serano, 2013). It behoves those reporting on non-binary gender to shift the discussion from these kinds of often intergenerational feminist/LGBT+ rights debates; to challenge the polarised right/wrong thinking that often pervades these kinds of debates more broadly (Barker, 2014); to represent the diversity of non-binary people and issues; and to celebrate the multiplicity of activisms which are currently happening, as evidenced from the review above.

At the same time, it would be helpful if this burgeoning non-binary movement took up Whittle's call to learn from its history and to also challenge any tendency to polarise into a false binary between 'us' (young, non-binary, right) and 'them' (old, binary, wrong). Intersectionality is another major challenge in this movement given that currently it is probably only safe for those of us occupying a high degree of cultural privilege to be 'out' publicly and/or in our work environments. This can mean that the main visible non-binary people end up being wealthy, highly educated, middle-class, white, often masculine-of-centre, and not visibly disabled. Coupled with the limited young, white, thin image of androgyny provided by the fashion industry, this can mean that non-binary people who do not fit this mould feel excluded from communities and that young people are presented with a very limited sense of what their options might be as a non-binary person—or whether this is even open to them. As with other movements, it's necessary for those in positions of power to do what they can to provide space, support, and visibility to more marginalised groups, and to step back where possible in order to allow more of a diversity of voices to speak.

There is also a lot to be done in terms of connecting up non-binary activism worldwide, campaigning within the UN universal human rights framework and the Council of Europe transgender resolution (which are inclusive of non-binary people), and learning from countries and cultures outside the west which are often further forward in terms of recognition of non-binary genders (for a review, see nonbinary.org, 2016b; see also Vincent & Manzano-Santaella, this volume). Finally, in terms of the strategies we employ, we would do well to heed the advice of our NB genderqueer elder 'Auntie Kate' to do what we need to do to become more comfortable in the world, but in so doing, "don't be mean."

At this point in the chapter, I would like to hand over to another long-term trans activist, writer, performer, and advice columnist, S. Bear Bergman, for a more personal reflection on one aspect of non-binary activism.

Non-binary Language

S. Bear Bergman

In the fall of 1993, I got into my first argument with a university professor about the validity of gender-nonspecific pronouns. It was the first of what would prove to be many, in the fullness of time. Freshly emboldened by the smartypantses with whom I spent hour upon hour chatting on the proto-internet, I explained to my professor that—in actual fact—there was nothing grammatically incorrect at all about my use of these tiny words. I smugly recited stanzas of Chaucer to prove the pedigree of hir and then held my head up and praised the activists of the Usenet who had invented ze to go with it. Finally, I offered up my cloth-bound, Routledge-imprinted copy of *Gender Outlaw* by Kate Bornstein, sprinkled with gender-nonspecific pronouns that I hoped to validate by their obviously serious serifs (and my identity right along with them). My professor, a second-wave feminist lesbian in linen separates, shook her head slowly. "Those are not words, and," she said, wrinkling her nose in evident distaste, "*that* is not a woman."

Two things struck me in the exchange, and continued to reverberate for decades: one, that this professor arrogated to herself the right to decide whether a word was "real" or not, and two, that she obviously felt this power extended to my gender identity (and that of many other people). The rejection of the word contained the rejection of the concept in general and me in particular. While I enjoy a little bit of dictionary fetishism as much as the next writer, her pronouncement (and the judgment it contained) was obviously not about the words themselves, but about her disapproval of the ideas they contained—underlined by her choice to disdain both the words with which Bornstein made it clear that ze did not, indeed, consider herself a woman and also hir gender presentation (including hir grandly goth-infused high-femme sartorial pronouncement). People who experienced themselves as neither men nor women, or as some combination thereof? Absolutely not, she said, putting her sensible Dansko clog down firmly on the subject.

(Twenty-two years later, the *Oxford English Dictionary* announced that it had included gender-nonspecific pronouns and honorifics, including the singular *they*, to their volumes. When I finished happy-dancing around the kitchen, I indulged at length in a fantasy in which I could buy, carefully highlight, and then mail several hundred volumes to university professors around the world, marking the page with an engraved card reading only "neener, neener, neener.")

For two decades, I campaigned on behalf of the words ze and hir with varying degrees of success. I used them as my personal pronouns and insisted that people use them for me in professional contexts, which meant negotiating that whoever introduced my talk had to read them out loud in front of students (and listening to the speaker make a tremendous performance of how uncomfortably they sat in their mouths, most of the time). I pressed newspaper and periodical writers and editors to use them in articles about me, with little success. I wrote entire books using gender-nonspecific pronouns, and after going ten rounds with my publisher that they really were real words and that I really did have the right to use them, fully half of the reviews my books received acknowledged that I preferred "invented" pronouns or "neologisms," and then proceeded to ignore them and use either a masculine or a feminine pronoun set to refer to me. This choice was recently, unpleasantly, echoed in a stunningly dismissive *New York Times* article about Sasha Fleischman of Oakland, California, a genderqueer-identified teenager who was set on fire while riding a city bus. Evidently not content to let physical violence stand on its own, the Grey Lady perpetrated its own linguistic violence with the following parenthetical:

(Telling Sasha's story also poses a linguistic challenge, because English doesn't offer a ready-made way to talk about people who identify as neither male nor female. Sasha prefers "they," "it," or the invented gender-neutral pronoun "xe." *The New York Times* does not use these terms to refer to individuals.) (Slater, 2015)

Let that sink in.

In her book *Epistemic Injustice*, British philosopher Miranda Fricker describes two particular kinds of oppression related to knowledge and language. One, she terms *testimonial injustice*, which she describes as the occasion upon which prejudice causes a person to be perceived as a less-credible or non-credible in their capacity as an informant. The other is *hermeneutical injustice*, where a person has no way to describe their experience because the conceptual frame doesn't exist yet due to their stigmatised or disempowered identity (Fricker, 2007). When I read her book, I nearly yelped in recognition of the experience so robustly described.

Making matters worse, it's not just the cisgender professors and copyeditors of the world who have fought me on every instance of gender-nonspecific pronouns. There are plenty of transgender- and/or transsexual-identified people who rail against the non-binary among us with just as much vigour. Their conviction, frequently offered at some volume, is that the idea of non-binary gender cheapens and distracts from their journey. That it's all right to move from the known and identified category of man to that of woman, or vice versa, but not to add additional categories and certainly, absolutely, not to say that the categories are flawed, optional, or even discussible. Though these people may have trans identities or medical histories, their relationship to gender is heteronormative and binary—there are two choices, world without end, amen.

This too, I would argue, is a matter of language as much as it is of anything else; in Fricker's parlance, trans people suffer a hermeneutical injustice and non-binary-identified people suffer it doubly. The cultural imagination about anyone who is not normatively gendered—trans bodies, trans identities, relationships, sex, geography, conflict, priorities—is substantially influenced by what we can talk or write about intelligibly. Since the modern conversation about gender identity is heavily medicalised, with brief and chilling digressions into legal terminology, so too are most of the words we have for ourselves and each other medical or legal legacy words, designed to reinforce the "normal" and shine the cold light of inquiry upon the Other. We have no playful language, no admiring language, no nuanced language, and no affirming language. Instead, we're stuck with obviously false dichotomies like "pre-op" and "post-op" that have led the entirety of cisgender humanity into the beliefs that (a) all transgender experience is defined in relationship to surgical procedures that have existed for roughly 75 years, even though transgender people have existed for millennia and I can prove that and (b) that there's a single-opportunity trans medical intervention, somewhat akin to the television show *Pimp My Ride*, where we enter looking one way and emerge entirely different and perhaps with a few things chromed.

What's more, the process of moving away from the medicalised language—which is full of terrible assumptions and worse ideas, but has the virtue of being somewhat familiar to even people who are quite distant from the topic—is messy and contested. There is no trans equivalent of the *Academie Français*, where a group of people meet, discuss, and decide what new words are actual words and what they mean. This leads to internal conflicts and heated debates among trans and non-binary people about what words are best to use, and because those debates are entirely decentralised, you could well find yourself using a word you learned in Chicago as respectful and appropriate and being told in Atlanta that you're using oppressive language and to get out. As an educator, I spend a lot of time explaining this: That trans communities have come to a place where we have the cultural agency, finally, to explain and describe our own experiences using our own language, and that while this is a messy and inconsistent process, it's also a pivotal (and frankly thrilling) moment in identity development. I have some sympathy for the well-meaning non-transgender people who desperately want to get the lingo right as an act of allyship with trans and non-binary people in this, but it's too important (and too exciting) to rush. If we're going to be able to eventually describe the specific, delicious, varied, and nuanced particulars of our non-normative bodies, experiences, and identities, it's going to take some time.

This is true even though the larger cultural imagination, with its limited and limiting understanding of trans and non-binary experiences, can't fathom what we might be taking our time on, or why it could be so important. Most people, especially the able-bodied, have rarely or never had the experience of having bodily experiences for which they have no word, or no word they can stand to use (masturbation stands alone as a frequent exception to this rule). The mental blank spot first gets filled with a placeholder, often "this" or sometimes "that." Then, maybe, it evolves to a shorthand code word, akin to a private joke or with one's self or the kind of idiolects married people inevitably develop over time. But eventually sometimes a moment arrives in which we hear a word for the very thing, and we see ourselves reflected in it. As a non-binary-identified person, that was also my experience of gender-nonspecific pronouns. The jolt of understanding, the dawning clarity of why I had shifted with discomfort when spoken about with feminine pronouns but had no especial desire to run to the warm embrace of masculine pronouns all but re-set my skeleton in my skin. Certainly, it shuffled the deck of my locution and dealt me a hand I had never previously understood to be a winner.

Where non-binary identities are concerned, the hermeneutical injustice that applied to trans people 20-odd years ago still rages, even though trans identities have seen some progress. For non-binary-identified (or, to use my current favourite term, *enby*) people, this is magnified by the fact that while most of everyone except Germaine Greer and Donald Trump are prepared to recognise that trans people do exist these days, the *enby* population is still struggling up that hill with our glitter in the one hand and our neckties in the other. These days, I deploy the word *enby*, which is just a pronunciation of the initials NB, for non-binary, with casual authority. I neither describe nor explain it unless asked. My part in the evolution of language around *enby* topic and identities is that I no longer engage in the kind of debates I used to about whether something is or is not a word; I know better now. Of course it's a word, I tell them, just like laser and radar are words, just like we used to fax things and now we Google them. I try to not even mansplain about it. But I'm wise to the tactic now, this thing of pretending to have some kind of high-minded linguistic objection to a new concept or idea being expressed in order to conceal a prejudice; I have experienced enough epistemic injustice to name it and stand up for myself and people like me as a legitimate expert on my own identity. With the cultural power I've concentrated as a public intellectual, a cultural worker, and—let us not forget—a white guy now, I have become stalwart in my assertions that people are and can be trusted to be, in the words of educator J Wallace Skelton, experts on themselves (Skelton, 2016). The smokescreen of being challenged about words has given way, and it develops that people are much more hesitant about saying "I think your identity is invalid because it challenges my beliefs about the world," than they ever were about saying "That's not a real word." Go figure.

(This becomes especially clear when an *enby* person uses the singular they pronoun, and suddenly there emerge strenuous objections to it from people who consistently misuse lie for lay and whose entire previous commitment to grammar expired sometime around the end of sentence diagramming in Grade 10. It would be funny if it weren't so exhausting and demoralising).

In the 22 years between when I started agitating on behalf of gender-nonspecific pronouns and when the OED joined the English language (already in progress) about gender-nonspecific pronouns—anointing them along with the gender-nonspecific honorific *Mx.* and the word *cisgender*—there has certainly been some progress in language. The cisgender imagination, and especially that of the gatekeepers of law, medicine, and language whose imprimatur so many things have previously required, is expanding and with it *must* go the language. Even the word cisgender—a word created and deployed by trans and *enby* people—now takes a fairly unchallenged place in academia at least (though it apparently upsets a certain subset of people whose gender privilege is so entrenched that they fuss and kick at being named with a word they didn't coin or choose, to whom I say: "Welcome.")

I begin to wonder at this point what will happen next—will the reality of our lives become so present and incontrovertible on the landscape of gender that refusal to use our words will become the last refuge of the bigot? Will there be a backlash against identity politics that causes cis people to insist that they don't see gender and therefore have no need to grapple with it anymore? How will forms, systems, data, and codexes of language evolve to capture the nuances of gender identity, and what new points of linguistic friction will each of those solutions inevitable produce? Even for cisgender folks, this is an exciting time indeed.

My friend Scott Turner Schofield, who used to be a performance artist and is now a soap opera actor (which he claims is a lateral move if ever there was one), tells a story I have long enjoyed about needing a particular tool while travelling in Costa Rica. He had no idea what it was called in Spanish, so he went to the hardware store intending to browse the available items and choose the thing he needed. But when he arrived, he discovered that the store was more or less a kiosk, and all of the tools were kept in the back, so a shopper was forced to ask for the thing they wanted and wait for it to be fetched back by the proprietor. Scott, stumped by this turn of events, produced in his limited Spanish the following request: I need the tool for turning with the top that's shaped like the church. After some puzzlement, the clerk laughed, nodded, and came back with what he needed: a Phillips-head screwdriver.

This is exactly, in many ways, where we find the language of trans—and especially non-binary—identities. Without knowing a word for what we need, we approximate based on what we think a conversation partner, reader, lover, doctor, or government official might be familiar with—and we stand and wait wearing our most cheerful and polite smiles while we hope that person will find themselves willing to do the extra work to understand. In the hopeful future, maybe the words of nuanced, descriptive, tender gendered language will be real in our mouths and on our screens. For now, we rely on goodwill and creativity to get the job done. The good news is, many of us have a lot of both.

Summary

To summarise this chapter, these are key points to keep in mind about non-binary activism:

* It is not a new thing: we can see the roots of current non-binary activism in the older trans, queer, and bisexual movements, and in some earlier forms of feminism, and it is important to open up intergenerational dialogue so that these groups can learn from one another.
* NB activism overlaps with academic work in its focus on conducting and reporting research with non-binary people so that activism can be grounded in persuasive evidence.
* NB activism often foregrounds campaigns for the rights of non-binary people to self-determine their gender and to have this accurately recorded, as well as campaigns for gender-inclusive language (pronouns, titles, etc.), and making public spaces gender neutral or non-binary inclusive.

- There is also a focus on awareness-raising and education to improve cultural understanding of gender, as well as the provision of support and resources for non-binary people themselves.
- It is important to include non-binary people in wider trans activist campaigns around areas such as prisons, asylum seeking, and—particularly—easy and inclusive access to medical services.
- Non-binary activism needs to be intersectional: recognising that non-binary experience intersects in key ways with race, class, age, geographical location, and all other aspects of identity and background.

Note

1. The Rotifer Project will be included in a case study in the forthcoming guidance AGENDA: A Young People's Guide on Making Positive Relationships Matter (Cardiff University, NSPCC, Welsh Women's Aid, supported by Children's Commissioner for Wales and National Assembly for Wales).

References

Note: Unless otherwise stated, all online materials were accessed at the time of writing in 2017

Action for Trans Health. (2016). *Falling Through the Cracks: Non-binary People's Experiences of Transition Related Healthcare*. Retrieved from http://www.actionfortranshealth.org.uk

All About Trans. (2016). *Gender Identity: Non-binary*. Retrieved from http://www.allabouttrans.org.uk/category/non-binary

Barker, M.-J. (2014, July 15). Trigger Warning: Trigger Warnings (Towards a Different Approach). *Open Democracy*. Retrieved from http://www.opendemocracy.net/transformation/meg-barker/trigger-warning-trigger-warnings-towards-different-approach

Barker, M.-J. (2015). *Activist/Academic Space Guidelines*. Retrieved from http://www.rewriting-the-rules.com/resources-2/activistacademic-space-guidelines

Barker, M.-J., & Lester, C. N. (2015). *Non-binary Gender Factsheet.* Retrieved from http://www.rewriting-the-rules.com/resources-2/non-binary-gender-factsheet

Barker, M.-J., Richards, C., Jones, R., Bowes-Catton, H., & Plowman, T. (2012). *The Bisexuality Report: Bisexual Inclusion in LGBT Equality and Diversity.* Milton Keynes, UK: The Open University, Centre for Citizenship, Identity and Governance.

Be: Non-binary. (2016). *Trans Support and Development in the North.* Retrieved from http://www.be-north.org.uk/events/be-non-binary-2016-04-17

Bem, S. L., & Lewis, S. A. (1975). Sex Role Adaptability: One Consequence of Psychological Androgyny. *Journal of Personality and Social Psychology, 31*(4), 634.

Bennet, J. (2016, January 30). She? Ze? They? What's in a Gender Pronoun? *New York Times.* Retrieved from http://www.nytimes.com/2016/01/31/fashion/pronoun-confusion-sexual-fluidity.html

Beyond the Binary. (2015, September 15). *#SpecificDetriment: What's Your Response?* Retrieved from http://www.beyondthebinary.co.uk/specificdetriment-whats-your-response

Beyond the Binary. (2016). *A Magazine for UK Non-binary People.* Retrieved from http://www.beyondthebinary.co.uk

Bornstein, K. (1994). *Gender Outlaw: On Men, Women and the Rest of Us.* New York: Routledge.

Bornstein, K., & Bergman, S. B. (Eds.). (2010). *Gender Outlaws: The Next Generation.* New York: Avalon Publishing Group.

Breaking the Binary. (2016). *Research and Journalism Project Exploring Non-binary Gender.* Retrieved from http://www.breakingthebinary.wordpress.com

Cambridge University Students' Union LGBT+ Campaign. (2016). *Recommendations: Toilet and Changing Facilities.* Retrieved from http://www.lgbt.cusu.cam.ac.uk/campaigns/think/recommendations

Carrigan, M., Gupta, K., & Morrison, T. G. (2013). Asexuality Special Theme Issue Editorial. *Psychology & Sexuality, 4*(2), 111–120.

Choudrey, S. (2016). *Inclusivity: Supporting BAME Trans People.* GIRES. Retrieved from http://www.gires.org.uk/assets/Support-Assets/BAME_Inclusivity.pdf

Elan-Cane, C. (2015, December 24). Non-gendered—Fighting for Legal Recognition. *The Huffington Post.* Retrieved from http://www.huffingtonpost.co.uk/christie-elancane/non-gendered_b_8870260.html

Fricker, M. (2007). *Epistemic Injustice: Power and the Ethics of Knowing.* New York: Oxford.

Galop. (2011). *Transphobia.* Retrieved from http://www.galop.org.uk/wp-content/uploads/2011/11/Transphobia-A4.pdf

Gendered Intelligence. (2013). *Non-binary Gender Identities: Information for Trans People & Allies.* Retrieved from http://cdn0.genderedintelligence.co.uk/2013/02/12/12-35-49-nonbinary0213.pdf

Genderqueer in the UK. (2016). *All the Information You Need to be Recognised Outside of the Gender Binary.* Retrieved from http://www.genderqueer-intheuk.wordpress.com

Gust, O. (2016, March 22). *Non-binary Performance Through Time.* Presentation to the Moving Beyond the Binaries of Sex and Gender Conference, University of Leeds.

Hines, S. (2016, March 22). *Trans Studies: Reflections and Advances.* University of Leeds Seminar.

House of Commons Women and Equalities Commission. (2016). *Transgender Equality.* HC390. Retrieved from http://www.publications.parliament.uk/pa/cm201516/cmselect/cmwomeq/390/390.pdf

Howitt, H. (2016). *Escape the Binary.* Retrieved from http://www.escapethebinary.com

Large, L. (2016, March 22). *Moving Towards a Non-binary Account of Gender Dysphoria.* Presentation to the Moving Beyond the Binaries of Sex and Gender Conference, University of Leeds.

Lees, P. (2016, March 10). Placing a Transgender Woman in a Men's Prison is a Cruel Punishment. *The Independent.* Retrieved from http://www.independent.co.uk/voices/comment/paris-lee-placing-a-trans-woman-in-a-mens-prison-is-a-cruel-and-unusual-punishment-a6923831.html

Lester, C. N. (2015, July 5). *"Genderfluidis the New Black": On the Media's Non-binary Moment.* Retrieved from http://www.cnlester.wordpress.com/2015/07/05/genderfluid-is-the-new-black-on-the-medias-non-binary-moment

Lester, C. N. (2016, March 22). *Challenging Canonicity: Musicology in Trans Activism.* Presentation to the Moving Beyond the Binaries of Sex and Gender Conference, University of Leeds.

Lorimer, S. (2016, January 14). Transgender Equality: Moving Away from Psychiatry. *The Huffington Post.* Retrieved from http://www.huffingtonpost.co.uk/dr-stuart-lorimer/transgender-equality-movi_b_8977614.html

Nestle, J., & Wilchins, R. A. (2002). *Genderqueer: Voices from Beyond the Sexual Binary.* New York: Alyson Publications.

NHS England. (2015). *Treatment and Support of Transgender and Nonbinary People Across the Health and Care Sector: Symposium Report.* National Health

Service Commissioning Board. Retrieved from http://www.england.nhs.uk/commissioning/wp-content/uploads/sites/12/2015/09/symposium-report.pdf

Nonbinary.org. (2016a). *Nonbinary Gender Visibility, Education and Advocacy Network*. Retrieved from http://www.nonbinary.org

Nonbinary.org. (2016b). *Recognition*. Retrieved from http://www.nonbinary.org/wiki/Recognition

Non-binary Inclusion Project. (2016). *Non-binary Inclusion Project*. Retrieved from http://www.nonbinary.co.uk

Non-binary London. (2016). *London Non-binary/Genderqueer Meet-up!* Retrieved from http://www.nonbinarylondon.tumblr.com

Non-binary Scotland. (2016). *Supporting Non-binary Gender People Living in Scotland*. Retrieved from http://www.nonbinaryscotland.org

Open Barbers. (2016). *Queer Friendly Hairdressing*. Retrieved from http://www.openbarbers.tumblr.com

Piercy, M. (1976). *Woman on the Edge of Time*. New York: Alfred A. Knopf.

Queen, C., & Schimel, L. (Eds.). (1997). *PoMoSexuals*. San Francisco, CA: Cleis Press.

Richards, S. E. (2014, February 19). Facebook's Gender Labeling Revolution. *Time Magazine*. Retrieved from http://time.com/8856/facebooks-gender-labeling-revolution

Saner, E. (2016, February 21). Caitlyn Jenner's Got Company: Meet Kate Bornstein, the One-Woman Whirlwind Who's Lived Many Lives. *The Guardian*. Retrieved from http://www.theguardian.com/tv-and-radio/2016/feb/21/kate-bornstein-interview-caitlyn-jenner-i-am-cait

Sanghani, R. (2015, December 14). Why the UK Should Ditch Male and Female Toilets for 'Gender-Neutral' Loos. *The Telegraph*. Retrieved from http://www.telegraph.co.uk/women/life/why-the-uk-should-ditch-male-and-female-toilets-for-gender-neutr

ScottishTrans.org. (2016). *UK Non-binary Survey*. Retrieved from http://www.scottishtrans.org/our-work/research/uk-non-binary-survey

Serano, J. (2013). *Excluded: Making Feminist and Queer Movements More Inclusive*. New York: Seal Press.

Skelton, J. W. (2016). *Transphobia: Deal with it and Become a Gender Transcender*. Halifax, Canada: Lorimer Publications.

Slater, D. (2015, January 29). The Fire on the 57 Bus in Oakland. *The New York Times Sunday Magazine*. Retrieved from http://www.nytimes.com/2015/02/01/magazine/the-fire-on-the-57-bus-in-oakland.html?_r=0

Stonewall. (2015). *Trans People and Stonewall*. London: Stonewall. Retrieved from http://www.stonewall.org.uk/sites/default/files/trans_people_and_stonewall.pdf.

Titman, N. (2014). *How Many People in the United Kingdom are Nonbinary?* Retrieved from http://www.practicalandrogyny.com

Tobia, J. (2015, August 31). I am Neither Mr, Mrs nor Ms but Mx. *The Guardian*. Retrieved from http://www.theguardian.com/commentisfree/2015/aug/31/neither-mr-mrs-or-ms-but-mx

Trans Media Watch. (2014). *Understanding Non-binary People: A Guide for the Media*. Retrieved from http://www.transmediawatch.org/Documents/non_binary.pdf

UK Lesbian and Gay Immigration Group. (2016, January 14). *Transgender Equality Inquiry: A 'Missed opportunity' for Trans Asylum Seekers*. Retrieved from http://www.uklgig.org.uk/?p=2101

Valentine, V. (2016, March 22). *Specific Detriment: A Survey into Non-binary People's Experiences in the UK*. Presentation to the Moving Beyond the Binaries of Sex and Gender Conference, University of Leeds.

Vincent, B., & Erikainen, S. (2016, March 22). *Moving Beyond the Binaries of Sex and Gender: Non-binary Identities, Bodies, and Discourses*. University of Leeds Conference, Conference booklet. Retrieved from http://www.gires.org.uk/pdfs/Conference%20Booklet.pdf

White, F. R. (2016, March 22). *Teaching Gender, Being Non-binary*. Presentation to the Moving Beyond the Binaries of Sex and Gender Conference, University of Leeds.

Whittle, S. (1996). Gender Fucking or Fucking Gender. In R. Ekins & D. King (Eds.), *Blending Genders: Social Aspects of Cross-Dressing and Sex-Changing*. Oxford: Psychology Press.

Wotever World. (2016). *Queer Performance and Events in London and Around Europe*. Retrieved from http://www.woteverworld.com

Further Reading

Barker, M.-J., & Scheele, J. (2016). *Queer: A Graphic History*. London: Icon Books.

Bornstein, K. (1994). *Gender Outlaw*. London: Routledge.

Bornstein, K., & Bergman, S. B. (Eds.). (2010). *Gender Outlaws: The Next Generation*. New York: Avalon Publishing Group.

Iantaffi, A., & Barker, M.-J. (2017). *Gender: A Guide for Every Body*. London: Jessica Kingsley.

Serano, J. (2013). *Excluded: Making Feminist and Queer Movements More Inclusive*. New York: Seal Press.

Wilchins, R. A. (1997). *Read My Lips: Sexual Subversion and the End of Gender*. Ann Arbor, MI: Firebrand Books.

4

Academic Theory

Jay Stewart

Introduction

This chapter sets out the key academic theories where non-binary gender identity, trans identities, and gender variance are covered.[1] Such theories are, no doubt, difficult to unpack from the historical and cultural contexts in which they are written. In addition to this, there are a multiplicity of academic fields where gender is discussed, as well as a wide variety of positions which each individual author is coming from. It is also important to keep the influences of political landscapes and grassroots activism coming from non-binary and other communities in mind. These drive changes in language, understanding, and concepts by drawing on, but also shaping, academic thinking.

This chapter will therefore endeavour to offer some context to the array of academic fields where non-binary gender is considered. My key questions are: *How is being non-binary understood across various fields of study?*

J. Stewart (✉)
Gendered Intelligence, London, UK

© The Author(s) 2017
C. Richards et al. (eds.), *Genderqueer and Non-Binary Genders*, Critical and Applied Approaches in Sexuality, Gender and Identity, DOI 10.1057/978-1-137-51053-2_4

And how does falling between or beyond a binary framework of gender (male/ female) get thought about and constructed through (and indeed between) various academic disciplines? Moreover: *How might non-binary/trans studies allow us to think about not only the study of non-binary/trans people but to critically think and 'know' in a non-binary/trans way?*

Whilst I note the various disciplines and the consequential inter-, multi-, or indeed trans-disciplinarity of the study of non-binary identities, gender variance, and transgender studies; I consider this chapter to be not only about an object of study (non-binary gender identities) but also about how—by considering non-binary gender identity—we might reconsider the thinking and cultural understanding of gender itself.

Like much gender-related academic work, I begin my chapter in the early nineteenth century. However, it's important to note that non-binary genders in their various manifestations, together with the variety of language used in describing them, have always been there (see Vincent and Manzano, this volume).

Sexology and a History of Gender Theories

Historically, theories of sex and gender were most notably considered within the medical field. Certainly with the emergence of psychoanalytic practice, this was where understandings of—and social dealings with—gender (and sexual) variance were offered more critical attention. Heterosexuality and the gender roles, identities, and expressions that were deemed 'normal' to those who were 'male' or 'female' were invisible and taken-for-granted, but sets of behaviours, desires, thoughts, and actions that were deemed 'different', 'other', or 'variant' began to be highly scrutinised and recorded. Indeed, it is the documentation through scientific, medical, and psychoanalytic texts—and specifically through case studies written by psychiatrists and sexologists—where we can come to understand concepts of gender variance in the early nineteenth century (e.g. Ellis & Pforzheimer, 1936; Krafft-Ebing, 1886).

In Vienna, medical psychiatry and the classifications of psychopathological sexual identities were first established in Von Krafft-Ebing's seminal *Psychopathia Sexualis* in 1886. Krafft-Ebbing focused on the 'invert' and homosexuality was noted as "contrary inverted sexual feelings". In Germany, Magnus Hirschfeld founded the Scientific Humanitarian Committee in 1897 and wrote *Geschlechtskunde* (*Sexual Knowledge*, 5 vols, 1926–1930). In addition, he established the Institute of Sexology, which was famously burnt down by the Nazis in 1933. Havelock Ellis's later book *Studies in the Psychology of Sex* (1936) considered 'congenital inverts', and this medical work, along with others, began the shifts towards thinking that homosexuality is "a sickness rather than a crime" (Hird, 2002, p. 579).[2] In his book *Science, Politics and Clinical Intervention*, Ekins writes:

> The early sexological tradition is notable for its emphasis upon systematic description of clinical pictures (nosography) and their classification (nosology), accompanied by etiological theorizing. In short, though the 'disease' status of sexual variations may be variously questioned by the early sexologists, the early sexologist tradition does follow the 'medical model' insofar as its collection of biographical and psychological data is followed by classification, diagnosis and etiological theorizing. (Ekins, 2005, p. 311)

These 'scientific' observations of 'inverts' were carried out through a scrutiny of looking and measuring. Sexologists would measure body parts, including skulls, and were known for carrying out autopsies on the dead in order *to know* something of this phenomenon through examining the materiality of the body (MacKenzie, 1994). The history of gender variance shows a complex entanglement between medical psychiatry and the emerging classifications of psycho-pathological sexual identities since the end of the nineteenth century.

It was a General Practitioner of Medicine, Cauldwell, who first issued the term 'transsexual' in reference to a FTM (female-to-male) patient he had worked with in 1949, who was seeking hormones and surgical treatment (Prosser, 1998; Stryker & Whittle, 2006). However, it was Harry Benjamin who popularised the term in 1953 in an article published in the *International Journal of Sexology* by distinguishing the 'transsexual' from the 'transvestite' (Benjamin, 1953). In addition, Harry Benjamin's *Transsexual Phenomenon* (1966) offered a more sympathetic approach to those who wished to undergo a 'sex change', and shifting understandings of trans from being 'psycho-pathological' to being a 'medical condition' or 'syndrome' played a crucial part in this. This distinction was, in part, achieved when, in 1967, Benjamin hypothesised that being trans was brought about endocrinologically (Ekins, 2005).

In terms of treatment, Benjamin's work marked the shift away from pure psychoanalysis and psychotherapy towards a multi-disciplinary medical approach with psychoanalysis working in conjunction with hormone administration as well as 'sex change' surgery. Working in Germany within the field of endocrinology, Benjamin collaborated with Austrian endocrinologist Eugen Steinach, who first isolated sex hormones and their effect. With a foot in both 'camps', Benjamin also worked with sexologist Magnus Hirschfield before moving to the United States before World War II, where he became a citizen and worked alongside Alfred Kinsey from 1949 onwards in San Francisco (Stryker & Whittle, 2006). Kinsey's idea of natural variation led to his famous cataloguing and counting of homosexual acts, as well as autoerotic and other sexual experiences outside (and inside) of the marital home. Kinsey's use of science and scientific methodologies gave validity to the subject of sex as a viable object of study in the sciences. By drawing on endocrinology and biological discourses, a particular respectability came with being trans that marked a shift from a 'psychosis' to a 'medical condition' model. But this shift was not an instant one, nor indeed have medical practitioners and institutes universally taken it up.

Psychiatrist Robert Stoller drew on the work John Money carried out at John Hopkins University in Baltimore, Maryland, in the late 1950s and early 1960s. It was here where a distinction between biological sex and social gender role was in some senses more firmly established. Despite drawing from psychoanalytic doctrines with regards to causation of being trans, Stoller did put forward a notion that there are 'biological substrates' to behaviour and in particular sexual behaviour and emerging gender identities. Stoller drew on Freud's study of infants where he stipulated that there is "evidence of a biological undercurrent upon which floated the postnatal, learned behaviour" (Stoller in Stryker & Whittle, 2006, p. 57).

This tension between the biological and the psychological in relation to causation was most poignantly exemplified through the case of John

Money and David Reimer in the early 1960s.[3] Money's central conceptual thread was that of 'gender neutrality' where babies are blank slates
on which (gender) identities are imposed and encultured upon the being.
When a circumcision damaged the penis of David Reimer at the age
of two, John Money and his team reassigned the child 'female'. As an
infant, Reimer's testicles were removed and feminising hormones were
administered. The argument here was that gender is constituted fully by
nurture, and life raised as a little girl would be ethical and predictable.
However, at the age of 14, Reimer rejected his female identity and began
living as a young man. During adulthood, David Reimer, following his
twin brother, took his own life. What has since been understood from
these tragic circumstances is an argument that gender identity formation
is not purely one of socialisation, but is possibly innate. This prompted
a set of biological theories about gender identity formation alongside the
growing themes of looking to hormonal and neurological aetiologies.[4]

Also working in the United States at the same time as John Money was
Harold Garfinkel, who pioneered the development of ethnomethodol-
ogy. This was a method which explored people's lived experience in the
context of the wider social world—and cultural understandings—around
them. Garfinkel's case study of 'Agnes'—a trans woman—carried out in
the 1960s was well documented, and it was through this case study that
the beginnings of understanding transsexualism as a form of intersex,
or having an intersex condition, came to pass. Robert Stoller, as well as
another sexologist Richard Green, saw 'Agnes' within clinical settings.
Richard Green had previously earned his medical doctorate in the early
1960s at John Hopkins University School of Medicine where John Money
was based, and eventually took his practice to the UK. Green, Stoller,
and Garfinkel agreed that 'Agnes' had a "rare intersex condition known
as testicular feminization syndrome" and she was referred for gender
reassignment surgery (the construction of a vagina) (Stryker & Whittle,
2006, p. 58). Garfinkel posited that expressing one's gender is a "managed achievement" (Stryker & Whittle, 2006, p. 58) and stipulated the
gender of 'Agnes' as a series of actions. This established understandings of
gender as 'doing' rather than 'being' (Papoulias, 2006, p. 231). From this
idea, social scientists Kessler and McKenna, who, like Garfinkel, utilised
ethnomethodological methods, drew on these texts to establish gender as

'performative' (Kessler & McKenna, 1978).[5] A concrete example of this has been captured in the film *The Danish Girl* which features the story of trans woman Lilly Elbe and her partner Gerda Wegener, where the film shows how we copy one another (not just trans people of course)—the way we sit, the way we walk, and so on. The film shows that at first learnt actions can be awkward or inauthentic, but through repeated acts can soon become 'natural' (Hooper, 2015).

Critiques of the 'Natural' and the Emergence of the 'Norm'

So far I have given a whistle-stop tour of the origins of understandings of gender variance within scientific and medical fields. For the sense of how these have developed and played out in recent psychological and psychiatric understandings, the reader is referred to the section on *Minds* below. What I wish to turn to now is to a critical engagement with such ways of knowing about gender variance. This critical literature—particularly queer theory—is notorious for being rather complex, so I will do my best to explain it simply and to provide further basic introductions in the further reading section for those who want to find out more.

Authorities often esteem scientific knowledge with its Galilean imperatives to prove a statement or to formulate a grand universal law. It was French philosopher Michel Foucault who crucially critiqued systems that treat these forms of knowledge as real objects that sit outside of our subjective interpretation (Foucault, 1995). He tells us how disciplines such as biology or psychiatry do not simply describe the distinctions between what is known (categories) and how it comes to be known (methodology), but are themselves technologies of power that position knowledge within elite bodies of specialist expertise (Foucault, 1976, 2003; Halberstam, 2011; Sedgwick, 1993). Foucault argued that there are no objective and universal truths, but that particular forms of knowledge and the ways of being that they engender, become 'naturalised', in culturally and historically specific ways (Sullivan, 2003).

There are many examples of how scientific thinking might have regarded itself as objective but in time reveals itself not to be. We can think of 'homosexuality', for instance, which has been deemed 'objectively' as a crime, a sickness, and an acceptable identity at different points in time. This shows how the cultural assumptions of those doing the studying impact on what is regarded as 'objective fact'.

What Foucault offered theoretically was that 'normal' behaviour is not a given, but is consequent to the set of values and moral order society sets and which are articulated by people, including medical practitioners. Many of the things people see as 'abnormal' in modern, Western society have not necessarily been considered as such in other times and places.[6] Establishing categorisations for 'abnormal behaviour' means to often draw on stereotypes, social expectations, and concepts of gender 'norms'. Of course, not conforming to gender norms is integral to non-binary existence.

Drawing on the work of Foucault, Judith Butler published *Gender Trouble* in 1990 and, like other critical and feminist writers at the time, she posed specific questions around the category of 'woman'.[7] Butler states that "The very subject of women is no longer understood in stable or abiding terms" (Butler, 1999, p. 4). Consequently, she asks, "Do the exclusionary practices that ground feminist theory in a notion of 'women' as subject paradoxically undercut feminist goals to extend its claim to 'representation'?"(Butler, 1999, p. 8). As the book wrestles with the political consequences of such exclusionary practices, Butler rests her query of what is a 'woman' not only in feminist theory but also in wider philosophical theories which ask 'who we are?', 'why we are who we are?', and how the law, or 'judicial power', plays a part in deeming an individual a 'legitimate' individual (Butler, 1999, p. 5). Butler raises some important considerations around how we become our 'selves', asking: what is it possible to become and what is not possible to become? What is already determined (I am who I am and there's nothing I can do about it) and where do we have choice (I am who I am because I have the freedom to pursue as such)?

Butler takes to task the ways in which sex and gender as concepts have been split for the purposes of forwarding the biology-is-not-destiny 'project' that gained momentum throughout the second wave of feminism. Feminism from the 1960s focused on the ways in which patriarchal culture enforced inequitable gender roles. These gender roles are not innate but are socially constructed in order to meet such patriarchal ends. We can think of expressions such as "a woman's place is in the home" to understand how a critical and political encounter with notions of domesticity attached to the role of women is no longer seen as a natural entity but as a social phenomenon. However, Butler shifts the thinking here by articulating that sex and the sexed body are also cultural as "We never experience or know ourselves as a body pure and simple, i.e. as our "sex", because we never know our sex outside of its expression of gender" (Butler, 1986, p. 39; in Hird, 2002, p. 585). Indeed, children can never understand themselves as male or female outside of all the cultural meanings and social roles that they have learnt around masculinity and femininity.

Butler confirms that the categories, the constructs, and even the nouns of 'male' and 'female' are to be understood in terms of their performativity and their repetitive acts; a repetition necessitated out of *a desire to be* constituted as being 'male' or 'female'. Drawing on Nietzsche, she stipulates that there is no 'I' prior to the acts of doing, no do-er behind the doing (Butler, 1999),[8] and continues:

> Gender is the repeated stylisation of the body, a set of repeated acts within a highly rigid frame that congeal over time to produce the appearance of substance, of a natural sort of being. (Butler, 1999, p. 63)

Put simply, if I were to walk down the street with a notable swagger, with a notable set of clothes, sporting a notable haircut, and talking in a notable voice that is socially noted and attributed to 'female-ness', or as feminine, it is the combination of these actions and codes that produce an appearance of 'being a woman' *as if* that was natural. Moreover, it is not only the singular act but the recognition of multiple repeated acts over time that make it seem as if being a woman is something essentialist and constant. Butler argues that, by considering gender (as a social construct) and as an effect that takes place after sex (the biological body), this makes it seem *as if* the sexed body is expressing gender in way that is 'natural'. A good way of thinking about this is to ask oneself: Why do we need to know the sex of a baby when it's born? The answer is that we need to know how to attribute gender performances to that baby. We will need to use certain pronouns, buy it certain clothes and toys, and paint its room a certain colour (see Fine, 2012, for more neuroscientific and psychological evidence for the impact of this on gender roles and expression). According to Butler, gender comes before sex and not the other way around (as suggested by John Money, for example). Butler states:

> The efforts to denaturalise sexuality and gender have taken as their main enemy those normative frameworks of compulsory heterosexuality that operate throughout the naturalisations and reification of heterosexist norms. (Butler, 1993, p. 11)

It is not then that sex comes prior to gender in terms of there already being a biological body, which is 'naturally' sexed and which consequently becomes cultured with gender—but rather that gender is prior to sex, as the performance of gender attributes an effect of an 'internal core' or 'substance' (Butler, 1990). For instance, a child that is assigned male at birth on account of having a penis might generate a host of assumptions and expectations from those around him that that child will enjoy and excel at football (a social norm certainly in particular cultures of the UK). Having a penis does not 'cause' a person to enjoy football; rather, it is the compelling and highly pressured social expectations around the child that 'produce' him as a person-who-plays-football and succumbs or fulfils these social gender norms.

The scene of subject production and establishing the sense of an internal core is never achieved outside of a regulatory framework. This is what Butler calls the Heterosexual Matrix (cf. Richards, 2017a): people are regarded as being either male or female, and as attracted exclusively to either males or females. One of the results of this is a 'queer project'— and arguably one that benefits non-binary people—which endeavours to demonstrate how sexuality, gender, and sex are not 'natural' but rather are socially constructed, and to expose the heterosexist norms involved.

To think through the performativity of sex can be difficult as it means to consider one's body not as an object or thing but as a site or place where meaning is produced. It is easier to think about fashion as being masculine or feminine and as something that shifts and changes. However, it is more tricky to think of body parts as *sites of meaning* that are also shifting as they are culturally and socially understood differently throughout history and place.

Queer Theory

Queer theory and politics necessarily celebrate transgression in the form of visible difference from norms. These 'Norms' are then exposed to *be* norms, not natures or inevitabilities. Gender and sexual identities are seen, in much of this work, to be demonstrably defiant definitions and configurations (Martin, 1996).

The political movement and critical discourse of 'Queer' emerged in the early 1990s, coming from Lesbian and Gay studies and feminist work and following such crucially important thinking as that of Michel Foucault and Judith Butler. Michael Warner tells us that "for both academics and activists, 'queer' gets a critical edge in defining itself against the normal rather than against the heterosexual" (Warner, 1994, p. xxvii). Queer theory works to deconstruct or undo 'compulsory heterosexuality' and homosexual prohibition and calls for the implementation of an 'opening up' (Butler, 1990, 1993; Sedgwick, 1994). Queer life and queer politics were to embrace hippy, punk, anarchist, anti-capitalist, anti-social 'rebel' identities that oppose the regulations of the Law. Queer was (and is) a calling for a working together to overthrow 'mainstream' thinking and articulate 'alternative' lifestyles.

In terms of gender, queer revisits and revises the categories of 'man' and 'woman' as fixed, essential single identities. As Sedgwick notably tells us:

> 'Queer' can refer to: the open mesh of possibilities, gaps, overlaps, dissonances and resonances, lapses and excesses of meaning when the constituent elements of anyone's gender, or anyone's sexuality aren't made (or can't be made) to signify monolithically. (Sedgwick, 1994, p. 8)

From these ways of thinking, trans and non-binary people have emerged as queer emblems who, through their very presentation of difference, expose the various constructs of gender, demonstrating opposition to the dominant forces of strict gender codes and practices, and revealing gender construction (Butler, 1991, 1993; Prosser, 1998). Notably, the realm of the visual in the form of art, photography, fashion, and performance (among others) has presented rich offerings to a cultural and critical encounter with gender expression.[9]

The Emergence of Transgender Studies

In order to consider the historical period that gave rise to the emergence of Transgender Studies, Susan Stryker maps out some of the activism that was taking place in the early 1990s in the United States. Sandy Stone's (1991)celebrated article, 'The Empire Strikes Back: A Posttranssexual Manifesto', called for refiguring transgender as resistant to a medicalised normalisation (Papoulias, 2006) and to expose transgender embodiment and histories as complex and resistant to overly simplistic ways of knowing about trans lives. Such stipulations were integral to the growing trans activist movement and engaged rigorously with the anti-trans radical feminism of the likes of Janice Raymond and Sheila Jeffreys.

In 1991, the Michigan Women's Music Festival expelled [trans] woman Nancy Jean Burkholder.[10] In addition, the anthology *Body Guards: the Cultural Politics of Gender Ambiguity* was published which, Stryker tells us, "Offered an early map of the terrain transgender studies would soon claim as its own" (Stryker & Whittle, 2006, p. 5).[11] In 1992, Leslie Feinberg's influential 'pamphlet' *Transgender Liberation: A Movement Whose Time Has Come* was published, in which the term *transgender* gained solidity and invoked solidarity to recognise the broad range of peoples who identified their gender as different to that which they were assigned at birth. *Transgender* as a term allowed for a range of choices of how an individual pursued and perceived their own gender identity which may or (importantly) may *not* include medicalised processes. In the same year, Transgender Nation formed in the region of San Francisco and trans activists were seen to become more mobilised. In 1993, the direct action group Transsexual Menace was founded by Rikki Anne Wilchins. Papoulias tells us:

> In the context of postmodern critiques of identity, transgender activism forged a challenge to hegemonic gender binaries and their naturalising force and invoked the possibility of fluid mobile and provisional enactments of gender. (Papoulias, 2006, p. 231)

Kate Bornstein's book *Men, Women and the Rest of Us* published in 1994 came out as she toured the university and community circuits with numerous performances which were autobiographical and drew on experience of being a *Gender Outlaw*. To mark the transgressive potential of transsexual people, Sally Hird drew on Bornstein. She tells us "Bornstein argues that transsexuals are not men or women, not because they are 'inauthentic' but because transsexuals, by their very existence, radically deconstruct sex and gender" (Hird, 2002, p. 589). Also in the early 1990s, activist Lou Sullivan presented openly as a gay trans man, inviting new debates around sexual orientations and practices that were not always heterosexual within transgender communities, despite the discourses—notably medical ones—which had implied this up to that point.

Narratives, testimonials, and autobiographies have also been central components of Queer Theory and Trans Studies, as well as of Feminism and Performance Studies (Duberman, 1997; Hart & Phelan, 1993; Martin, 1996; Phelan, 1993). Debates around sincerity, authenticity, and subjectivity have been critical for engagement, particularly with the autobiographical work of minority identities and 'otherness'. This has come from phenomenological ideas that privilege experience and being in the world and which have become central to a political and theoretical exploration of female/feminine, queer, black, disabled, and indeed trans, lives. Much queer writing has been concerned with autobiographical work. Queer writing commits itself not only to the critical attention of queer subjectivities, but to consideration of the productive possibilities of challenging and reframing heteronormative knowledge productions (Foucault, 1976; Sedgwick, 1994; Warner, 1994).

As queer theory and feminism—mainly through the work of Butler—established the beginnings of transgender studies and a shift or rise in trans activism, Jay Prosser expressed his own troubled sense of transgender bodies being too dominant a visual trope for queer theory—an image that exemplifies and exposes the mainstream cultural production of gender norms through visual means (Prosser, 1998). This is particularly problematic for Prosser when "such perspectives elide the materiality of trans bodies and the practices of embodiment which constitute trans experience in their specificity" (Papoulias, 2006, p. 232). In short, Prosser returns a certain 'seriousness' to the trans subject where queer theory has produced trans bodies as a site in which to play or 'fuck' with gender.

For non-binary people, there is a need to offer some reflection around the ways in which theoretical applications to non-binary and gender variant individuals (and gender diversity more broadly) are beneficial to our trans communities. Prosser is saying that it is all very well that gender non-conforming bodies and identities might expose the mechanisms of gender normativity itself, but there are some very real material consequences for non-binary individuals who navigate and negotiate prejudice and inequities in everyday life. The materiality of everyday life and the possibility of day-to-day existence as a non-binary person contrasts with the ways in which queer theory has remained quite abstract in its theory and has not given due attention to the political work at hand endeavouring to improve people's lives.

Prosser also points towards how the embodiment of gender variance locates itself (and is located in) a variety of knowledge fields that offer rather contradictory meanings. For instance, whilst in some knowledge fields trans has located itself as a postmodern subject—multiple in its narratives, fluid, and socially constructed—in other knowledge fields trans posits the sexes of 'male' and 'female' as natural, and supports subjectivities as fixed and stable entities within discourses of the biological (Prosser, 1998; cf. Richards 2017b).

Recent Directions

At the beginning of the foreword of the *Transgender Studies Reader* published in 2006, Stephen Whittle makes clear the extent to which transsexual and transgender subjects have become a focus for discourse across an array of knowledge fields and disciplines throughout the 1990s (Stryker & Whittle, 2006). In the introduction to the same reader, Susan Stryker marks a distinction where, prior to the 1990s, trans people were the object of study (transgender phenomena), but following this surge in attention, an emerging rise in the numbers of trans people themselves taking up the positions of writer, researcher, and academic marked "a new wave of transgender scholarship" (Stryker & Whittle, 2006, p. 1). Importantly, such trans scholars offered their own and other transgender lives, identities, and culture as central to the focus of their investigations and critical thinking.

Prior to 1990s, much discourse attributed to a 'trans epistemology' also centred around a taxonomy of sex and gender through the fields of psychology and the medicalisation of transsexualism. In an article 'For a Sociology of Transsexualism', Myra J. Hird calls for a "...displacement of psychology with sociology" (Hird, 2002, p. 578) in order to reorient theories of transsexualism and to "advanc[e] the need for a distinctly sociological approach to this particular identity" (ibid.). Building on the work of Garfinkel, as well as Kessler and McKenna, Hird acknowledges how the field of sociology emphasises the social construction of gender.

Hird advocates an understanding of transsexualism within society rather than holding centrally the individual psyche. Drawing on Moi (1999), Hird also claims a need to draw more substantially on phenomenological frameworks and theories of embodiment to stipulate gender as a set of histories and experiences. Certainly Hird notes that "transsexualism has been mostly theorised from medical and psychiatric perspectives" (Hird, 2002, p. 581). However, Hird attempts to disrupt the dominance that the field of psychology and psychoanalysis has had over trans identities. Papoulias on the other hand suggests that more psychoanalytic work can be done around trans experiences as a way to "invest our bodies with meaning" (Papoulias, 2006, p. 232). Whilst Papoulias concurs that "psychoanalytic readings of transgender experiences have been roundly denounced by transgender activists as productive of pathologising discourse" (ibid.); she also asserts that the field of psychoanalysis may still have its uses, stating:

> Psychoanalytic readings of transgendered subjectivity remind us of the unconscious phantasies which participate in our embodiment... [and] they propose that embodiment, whether transgender or not, is a process that no singular language (be it that of neurobiology, phenomenology, or indeed psychoanalysis itself) can fully translate. (Papoulias 2006, pp. 232–233)

Given these competitive dynamics to the ways in which trans subjectivities become known, Transgender Studies are a growing academic field which not only examines transgender communities as 'minority' communities but also engages in wider interrogations of how gender identities and subjectivities are produced (Stryker & Whittle 2006). Transgender Studies are integral to the politics, activism, and scholarly writing on feminism, sexuality studies, queer theory, and the Intersex Movement. Importantly, Transgender Studies, by their very interdisciplinary nature, wrestle with ideas and discourses held within the different fields and disciplines of sociology, history, cultural studies, and other arts and humanities field; as well as the sciences of biology, biochemistry, neurology, psychology, and psychiatry. This multidisciplinarity produces a rich, but often contradictory, set of knowledge frameworks that do not easily cohere in any single or 'general' idea of sex, gender, and what it means *to be trans*. Indeed, the different knowledge fields in which trans may be located conceptualise trans in particular ways pertaining to the various conventions and norms of the particular field or discipline.

For non-binary identities, it is helpful to expose and reflect on the academic understandings of gender in its broadest sense as suitably messy and contradictory. Non-binary gender identities trouble normative ideas of sex and gender, but they also reveal the ways in which meanings of sex and gender are conceptualised.

The emergence of Transgender Studies as its own academic area is still in its early stages. For non-binary individuals, emerging collectives, and the activism that is currently gaining momentum and visibility (see Barker & Bergman, this volume), more academic studies of non-binary gender are most necessary. What the scholarship of gender has shown so far is the constraint, and arguably violence, attributed to gendered lives through an allocation of being *either* male *or* female. The limitations and restrictions that abound from such an assignment of sex at birth are damaging to many people, including non-binary people. Non-binary lives, however, are offering a perspective that is powerful, rich, and exciting; indeed, non-binary people are carving out a pathway of possibilities that are currently relatively unexplored, they/we are the avant-garde of gendered existence which is shifting the landscape of gendered possibilities.

Summary

- In the nineteenth and early twentieth centuries, gender variance was often taken as a sign of biological sexual 'deviance'. Subsequently, gender was regarded as an entirely learnt social role by John Money and his colleagues.
- Early sociological work on trans shifted the understanding to one of gender performativity. According to Butler, normative genders are written onto bodies through repeated performance. Neither social gender nor biological sex is 'natural', and they are inextricably linked.
- Queer theory challenges the idea that there are hierarchical binaries of sexuality and gender (gay/straight and male/female) and the concept of fixed, essential identities, creating space for non-binary genders.
- Transgender studies developed out of trans activism and challenged the ways in which trans people had been pathologised in medical discourses; and celebrated as inevitably transgressive in queer discourses. They shifted the focus to the diverse lived experiences of trans people.
- Academic work on non-binary people similarly needs to chart their diverse lived experiences and to take account of the material realities of living non-binary in a binary gender world.

Notes

1. There are differences of views regarding the relationship between non-binary gender identity and trans identity. For the main part identifying one's self as non-binary forms part of the varied constellation of identities within the diverse trans community. Some non-binary people have wished to distinguish their identity from the trans community, mainly because of poor experiences, or feeling unacknowledged or unaccounted for from within this. The term *trans* (or sometimes *trans**) has been used to posit a very wide and all-encompassing understanding of the diverse trans communities, specifically regarding non-binary inclusion. *Gender variance* is a term that describes more a set of behaviours rather than categorising an identity in and of itself and for this reason can be productive. In addition, gender variance is often used to describe the behaviours of children and young people who are not currently identifying themselves as non-binary, trans, or using other words

more commonly understood as identity categories. There are medical connotations to the expression however, as it does have a history within medical discourse. For the purposes of this chapter I mean to fully include the identity of *non-binary* within the term *trans*.

2. Hird also writes about the accustomed sexism and patriarchal framings of such investigations on these people as effeminacy and female identities on male bodiedness was regarded as a 'failure', whilst any expressions of masculinity or male identities on female bodiedness were considered by von Krafft-Ebing as proficient individuals (Hird, 2002).

3. A documentary made as part of the Horizon Series in the UK called the *The Boy Who Was Turned into a Girl* (2002 Editor: Andrew Cohen BBC2 UK) focused on this story.

4. This also raises concerns around the ways in which medical practitioners intervene on the body—specifically in terms of gender identity—or indeed where a person may look to the medical world for solutions to living in a body whose gender/sex signifiers are so significantly compromised (Butler, 2001, 2004). In addition to the debates these bring to Transgender Studies, campaigners for the rights of people with intersex conditions have also drawn upon the case to challenge the medical and surgical interventions being made upon babies that were born with 'ambiguous genitalia' (Sterling, 2000). See also: http://www.isna.org/faq/reimer.

5. In the foreword to Garfinkel's essay *Passing and the Managed Achievement of Sex Status in an "Intersexed" Person*, published in *The Transgender Studies Reader*, Stryker and Whittle tell us that the added 'twist' in the story of 'Agnes' was that she did not disclose to her doctors the fact that she was self-medicating with her mother's female hormones for fear that she would not be admitted for genital surgery.

6. *See* https://whatmakesyourgender.wordpress.com/the-project/about-the-project/establishing-the-norm/ WHO AM I? *Hacking into the Science Museum project delivered by Gendered Intelligence with the Science Museum. The website states: "Before the 1830s, normal was a mathematical term, referring to a particular type of angle. In the 1830s, it became increasingly used in statistics, with the "normal distribution" a new way of measuring populations. It was agreed that most characteristics would fit on a bell curve. It wasn't until scientists began to apply this idea to health and illness that the term 'normal' began to be seen as desirable. Average blood pressure, for example, was considered to be healthy, and those with high or low blood pressure would require treatment to try and bring them closer to the norm. Applying this idea to all sorts of social characteristics led people to see 'normal' as being both good and healthy, rather than simply meaning the average of the population."*

7. See Wittig (1992) and de Lauretis (1989).
8. Butler is quoting Nietzsche's 1887 *On the Genealogy of Morals*.
9. Examples include the work of 'gender terrorist' and queer photographer Del la Grace Volcano (www.dellagracevolcano.com) and Sarah Deragon's Identity Project (www.identityprojectsf.com). Also in popular culture there are a whole raft of icons, including the late David Bowie, Annie Lennox, and Boy George. Also see the writings of Jack Halbastam.
10. See Burkholder (1993).
11. See Epstein and Straub (1991).

References

Benjamin, H. (1953). Transvestism and Transsexualism. *International Journal of Sexology, 7*, 12–14.

Benjamin, H. (1966). *The Transsexual Phenomenon*. New York: The Julian Press.

Bevan, T. (Producer), & Hooper, T. (Director). (2015). *The Danish Girl* [Motion Picture]. England: Working Title Films.

Bornstein, K. (1994). *Gender Outlaw: On Men, Women and the Rest of Us*. New York: Routledge.

Burkholder, N. J. (1993). *Michigan Women's Music Festival. Transsisters: The Journal of Transsexual Feminism, 2*(November/December), 4.

Butler, J. (1986). *Variations on Sex and Gender: Beauvoir, Wittig, and Foucault. Praxis International, 5*(4), 505–516.

Butler, J. (1990). *Gender Trouble: Feminism and the Subversion of Identity*. New York: Routledge.

Butler, J. (1991). Imitation and Gender Insubordination. In D. Fuss (Ed.), *Inside/Out: Lesbian Theories, Gay Theories*, (pp. 13–31). New York: Routledge. Reprinted in Sara Salih (Ed.). (2004). *The Judith Butler Reader* (pp. 119–137). Malden, MA: Blackwell.

Butler, J. (1993). *Bodies that Matter: On the Discursive Limits of 'Sex'*. New York: Routledge.

Butler, J. (1999). *Gender Trouble: Feminism and the Subversion of Identity* (2nd ed.). New York: Routledge.

Butler, J. (2001). *Doing Justice to Someone: Sex Reassignment and Allegories of Transsexuality. GLQ, 7*(4), 621–636.

Butler, J. (2004). *Undoing Gender*. New York: Routledge.

Cohen, A. (Ed.). (2002). *The Boy Who Was Turned Into a Girl* [Television Programme]. London: BBC.

Duberman, M. (Ed.). (1997). *Queer Representations: Reading Lives, Reading Cultures*. New York: New York University Press.

Ekins, R. (2005). Science, Politics and Clinical Intervention: Harry Benjamin, Transsexualism and the Problem of Heteronormativity. *Sexuality, 8*(3), 311.

Ellis, H., & Pforzheimer, C. (1936). *Studies in the Psychology of Sex* (1st ed.). New York: Random House.

Epstein, J., & Straub, K. (1991). *Body Guards: The Cultural Politics of Gender Ambiguity*. New York: Routledge.

Fine, C. (2012). *Delusions of Gender*. London: Icon Books.

Foucault, M. (1976). *The History of Sexuality* (1st ed.). Paris: Éditions Gallimard.

Foucault, M. (1995). *Discipline and Punish: The Birth of the Prison* (A. Sheridan, Trans.). New York: Vintage.

Foucault, M. (2003). *Society Must Be Defended: Lectures at the College de France, 1975–1976* (D. Macey, Trans.). New York: Picador.

Halberstam, J. (2011). *The Queer Art of Failure*. Durham, NC: Duke University Press.

Hart, L., & Phelan, P. (Eds.). (1993). *Acting Out: Feminist Performances*. Ann Arbor: University of Michigan Press.

Hird, M. J. (2002). For a Sociology of Transsexualism. *Sociology, 36*(3), 577–595.

Kessler, S. J., & McKenna, W. (1978). *Gender: An Ethnomethodological Approach*. Chicago: University of Chicago Press.

Krafft-Ebing, R. (1886). *Psychopathia Sexualis* (1st ed.). Germany.

Lauretis, T. (1989). *Technologies of Gender: Essays on Theory, Film and Fiction*. Bloomington: Indiana University Press.

Mackenzie, G. O. (1994). *Transgender Nation*. Bowling Green, OH: Bowling Green University Popular Press.

Martin, B. (1996). *Femininity Played Straight: The Significance of Being Lesbian*. New York: Routledge.

Moi, T. (1999). *What Is a Woman? And Other Essays*. Oxford: Oxford University Press.

Papoulias, C. (2006). Transgender. *Theory, Culture & Society, 23*, 231–233.

Phelan, P. (1993). *Unmarked: The Politics Of Performance*. New York: Routledge.

Prosser, J. (1998). *Second Skins: The Body Narratives of Transsexuality*. New York: Columbia University Press.

Richards, C. (2017a). Starshine on the Critical Edge: Philosophy and Psychotherapy in Fantasy and Sci-Fi. *Journal of Psychotherapy and Counselling Psychology Reflections, 2*(1), 17–24.

Richards, C. (2017b). *Trans and Sexuality—An Existentially-Informed Ethical Enquiry with Implications for Counselling Psychology* [Monograph]. London: Routledge.

Sedgwick, E. K. (1993). *How to Bring Your Kids Up Gay. Social Text, 29, 18–27.*
Sedgwick, E. K. (1994). *Tendencies.* London: Routledge.
Sterling, A. F. (2000). *Sexing the Body: Gender Politics and the Construction of Sexuality.* New York: Basic.
Stone, S. (1991). A Posttransexual Manifesto. In J. Epstein & K. Straub (Eds.), *Body Guards: The Cultural Politics of Gender Ambiguity.* New York: Routledge.
Stryker, S., & Whittle, S. (2006). (De)Subjugated Knowledges: An Introduction to Transgender Studies. In S. Stryker & S. Whittle (Eds.), *The Transgender Studies Reader.* New York: Routledge.
Sullivan, N. (2003). *A Critical Introduction to Queer Theory.* Edinburgh: Edinburgh University Press.
Warner, M. (Ed.). (1994). *Fear of a Queer Planet: Queer Politics and Social Theory.* Minneapolis: University of Minnesota Press.
Wittig, M. (1992). *The Straight Mind and Other Essays.* Boston: Beacon Press.

Further Reading

Barker, M.-J. & Scheele, J. (2016). *Queer: A Graphic History.* London: Icon Books.
Sullivan, N. (2003). *A Critical Introduction to Queer Theory.* New York: New York University Press.
Stryker, S., & Whittle, S. (2006). *The Transgender Studies Reader.* London: Taylor & Francis.
Wilchins, R. A. (2004). *Queer Theory, Gender Theory: An Instant Primer.* New York: Alyson Publications Inc.
Weeks, J. (2009). *Sexuality.* London: Routledge.

5

Law

Rob Clucas and Stephen Whittle

Introduction

This chapter[1] discusses the interface between people with non-binary gender identities (including genderqueer, gender-fluid, gender non-conforming, and gender variant identities) and law. The focus here is predominantly on the law of England and Wales, with references to other jurisdictions and international developments as a comparison. Of significance to current English and Welsh law, and to any jurisdiction contemplating reform of gender identities, is an examination of the recent Inquiry of the UK Parliament's Women and Equalities Committee into Transgender Equality, discussed further below. This chapter evaluates how the law comprehends, recognises, and provides protection (or not)

R. Clucas (✉)
University of Hull, Hull, Yorkshire, UK

S. Whittle
Manchester Metropolitan University, Manchester, Greater Manchester, UK

© The Author(s) 2017
C. Richards et al. (eds.), *Genderqueer and Non-Binary Genders*, Critical and Applied Approaches in Sexuality, Gender and Identity, DOI 10.1057/978-1-137-51053-2_5

for people with identities outside the male/female binary; and highlights the significant mismatch between the actuality of these identities and their acknowledgement in the practical interactions of daily life.

Non-binary?

The term *non-binary* is used as an all-encompassing name for those people whose gender identities fall outside the dominant societal gender binary.[2] It is impossible to discuss non-binary gender identities in the singular; they are a complex series of identities both within and outside of the understanding of gender being binary, that is boy and man, girl and woman. Some argue that the phrase *non-binary* excludes trans identities that are binary-oriented, such as *trans man* and *trans woman*. However, to do so is short sighted:

> To encounter the transsexual body, to apprehend a transgendered consciousness articulating itself, is to risk a revelation of the constructedness of the natural order. Confronting the implications of this constructedness can summon up all the violation, loss, and separation inflicted by the gendering process that sustains the illusion of naturalness. (Stryker, 1994, p. 93)

Purging structural systems of that illusion of gender naturalness has been at the core of trans activism, as articulated by trans academics as they created the field of Trans theory. The 1990s saw transsexual[3] and transgender[4] (trans) scholars and activists lead the discussion in which the constructed nature of gender difference and the limits of its mental spaces were acknowledged and challenged, effectively asking whether there is anything at all natural about having two genders:

> One answer to the question 'Who is a transsexual?' might well be 'Anyone who admits it.' A more political answer might be; 'Anyone whose performance of gender calls into question the construct of gender itself'. (Bornstein, 1994, p. 121)

The idea of a third (or fourth, or fifth, ...) gender may have been rejected by many courts[5] as the judiciary dismissed the claims that trans people brought for recognition of their particular gender identity; yet the very fact that trans people brought those claims before the courts has proliferated the visibility of their transgressive gender performances. It was the activism of trans people and their willingness to demonstrate the reality of transgressing gender boundaries; by challenging the limitations of law, and exploring their experiences through the media, that created an awareness of the fluidity of socially constructed gender boundaries. They made vulnerable the model of binary genders using new methods of social and political changes, effectively ensuring death by the Internet. The result:

> A trans identity is now accessible almost anywhere, to anyone who does not feel comfortable in the gender role they were attributed to at birth, or has a gender identity at odds with the labels 'man' or 'woman' credited to them by formal authorities. (Whittle, Foreword, in Stryker & Whittle, 2006)

Bornstein (1994) referred to those who cannot comprehend a world in which there are a plurality of genders as the 'Gender Defenders.' Amongst these, 1970s' radical feminists were the loudest protesters at the gender transgressions of trans people (Raymond, 1979). They claimed they were the ones promoting true gender transgressions; but their insistence on the uniqueness of the biological category of woman would undermine their arguments. Their voices still exist, but have sounded increasingly isolated and shrill. Some wrote to the recent Inquiry of the UK Parliament's Women and Equalities Committee into Transgender Equality, to oppose access to women's facilities for [trans] women. They brought forward reactionary arguments which refuse to recognise any sense of gender fluidities as embodied by the trans community, instead continuing to claim that trans lives cause oppression by upholding gender stereotypes (Jeffreys, 2015).

From the 1950s to early 1990s, gender identity clinics were the only places to provide any support to people uncomfortable in their assigned gender. Some clinicians working in the field had narrow views of men's and women's social and sexual roles and undoubtedly promoted, and in some cases insisted on, stereotypical gender role behaviour by their trans patients. Many will have felt obliged to conform to what was at the time seen as common sense knowledge. However, when trans man Lou Sullivan came out as gay in the late 1980s, he effectively gave many trans people permission to re-evaluate their sexuality and the identity their 'gender' gave them (Zagria, 2013). Since the publication of Sandy Stone's *The Empire Strikes Back* (1992), trans activists and scholars responding to her call to reclaim our histories have become auto-ethnographers, engaging with and challenging the view that gender is only binary. They have created their own academic events and conferences, and worked within organisations like the World Professional Association for Transgender Health (WPATH) (Fraser, 2015) and the APA (2015), insisting upon modernisation within the clinical frameworks that provide medical support for trans people. The recognition of gender pluralities is written large now within the *International Standards of Care for the Health of Transsexual, Transgender, and Gender-Nonconforming people* (Coleman et al., 2012).

All this has meant that paradoxically, on the one hand, transgender and transsexual people are increasingly now seen as having ordinary, if moderately rare, aspects of gender identity development—yet at the same time, more of them are declaring a more complex, non-binary gender identity. Undoubtedly, some trans people do see themselves as having a gender which sits on one or the other side of a gender divide, but many working with the trans community would say that this is an increasingly rare presentation of personal gender knowledge, as can be seen in the written evidence sent to the recent UK Inquiry into Transgender Equality (Women and Equalities Committee, 2015—discussed further below). A significant number of submissions came from people who had 'commenced permanently living in their preferred gender role,' but only in the sense that their 'preferred gender role' is one understood by cisgender people, not by the person themselves. They might appear as trans, but their personal understanding of their gender identity is far more complex. More than 15 % of submissions came from people referring to themselves as having a non-binary gender identity. This group was not necessarily a younger group, but crossed the age range, reflecting the development of complex gender understandings that many older trans people have already arrived at, through discussion, study, activism, and life experience:

If somebody asked me for an easy answer I would say I was born a boy it was just that nobody could see it [...] It is obviously much more complex than that. [...] you have a positioning which sort of shifts just slightly on one side of the scale. In other words [...] you're not a feminine woman, [...] but you're not actually a man at that point [...] then you sort of step over that line, [...] but you don't quite make it into full manhood, ever. (Stephen Whittle speaking in Self and Gamble, 2000, p. 47)

And yet, this is not a complete story. A plurality of gender identities still excludes some. Christie Elan-Cane says, "I really wish that people would not refer of [sic] my non-gendered identity as my 'gender identity'. I am non-gendered. I have a core identity that is as real and valid as the core identity of any gendered person but it is not a gender identity. It is an identity" (Elan-Cane, 2011). Elan-Cane's position is that to talk of per[6] as having a non-binary gender misses the point completely. Elan-Cane is a person who does not equate their personal sense of being as having any sort of gender. Referring to per as having a non-binary, or non-gendered identity equates per's sense of selfhood still within the context of gender, yet per lives outside of, and without gender (for anthropological perspectives on gender pluralities, see Waldemar Bogoras in Williams, 1988).

For many people with non-binary identities, or identities outside of any genders—whether trans or not—this is the real problem. Our social and legal structures insist that gender is binary. Many trans and non-trans people frequently, and for very good reasons, opt for safety over activism in their lives; meaning conformity to a pretence. Having spent their childhood pretending to be of their assigned gender, in adulthood pretending to be of another gender is not that hard if it ensures employment, housing, and healthcare. However, that does not mean to say they are content, as was clearly seen in the many submissions to the recent UK Parliamentary Inquiry (Women and Equalities Committee, 2015).

In the last 12 years, the UK has seen the implementation of the Gender Recognition Act (2004), The Civil Partnership Act (2004), the Equality Act (2010), and the Marriage (Same Sex Couples) Act (2013); and increasingly lesbian, gay, bisexual, and trans people are aware of their legal rights. So many people with non-binary gender identities submitted evidence to the Parliamentary Inquiry because, trans or not, they want not to merely have rights, but also to have their rights afforded recognition in law. There is many an equivocation that can be made to survive, but equivocations will ultimately produce problems. For a recent example at the birth registration of a child, the birth mother found himself referred to as the father, or partner—as on paper only the legally recognisable 'woman' in a relationship can be the child's mother, even though she was not the person to give birth. It seems the only way round is for the birth mother to become a surrogate mother, then he can give the child to be jointly adopted by his partner and himself as if they were step parents. The tangled web of inadequate law is never conducive to happy families!

Non-binary-Gendered Lives and the Legal Interface

In order to highlight these inadequacies, we discuss the law as it relates to England and Wales, with occasional reference to other jurisdictions to highlight significant differences. Further, by discussing international and domestic developments, it is possible to see how there is now at least an inkling in some law that gender identities are much more complex than previously imagined. Looking at a range of examples of the law-related interactions non-binary people face on a regular basis, these are essentially instances where non-binary identities or behaviours disrupt the assumptions society makes about gender assignment—how many genders there are, and what qualifies a person as a particular gender. These interactions are jarring, disruptive, and potentially threatening to the person with a non-binary gender identity. Their negotiation of everyday life brings them, repeatedly, into conflict with society's preconceptions and prescriptions.

Name

At birth, parents register a chosen first (middle) and last name for their child. Most people will continue to use this name for all purposes; however, some will change their name for a variety of reasons. Women often now choose to use their natal last name for professional purposes, and their spouse or partner's last name for family matters. The name given at birth will be shown on a person's birth certificate, naturalisation certificate, and so on, and this will not usually change. Exceptions are when a child's name is changed on an adoption certificate, or when a child's 'sex' has been incorrectly determined at birth, or when a trans person is issued a new birth certificate after obtaining legal recognition of their acquired (preferred) gender.

Change of Name in the UK

In the UK, unlike many other European states, a person may change the name assigned at birth as often as they wish, though it will remain on their birth certificate unless they apply for legal gender recognition. There are very few restrictions on what a formal change of name may be, so long as a new name is not for the purposes of passing-off or deception. The Registrar General will only refuse names, at birth registration, which cannot exist (because they cannot be said) or which are obscene. The Registrar cannot refuse (though they may so advise) to register the name, for example, of a child given all of the surnames of the Manchester United football team. This means that gender-neutral names are easily achieved in the UK.

The law allows a change of first, middle, and last (sur)names simply through custom and practice (i.e. without undergoing any legal process), unless the person is under the age of 16, when a declaration of consent from all those with parental responsibility is required, or a court order. However, in reality, many institutions including government departments, frequently, but incorrectly, insist upon evidence of a formal process to record a change of name. Most people will use a self-typed statutory declaration of name change, or if trans, a declaration of name and gender change. The declaration requires notarisation—a five-minute solicitor's appointment which currently costs £7 (2015). Deed polls are often accepted as proof of name change, at least in some areas of the UK, but may also require notarisation. Furthermore, the details on a deed poll including former names alongside new names have to be published in the *London Gazette*. As such these are inappropriate for trans people who wish to retain control over their privacy.

Formal name change documents can be used to change most personal paperwork, including a passport, driving licence, bank account, and so on, and thus provide everyday evidence of a person's new name, without indicating that this name is not the name originally given. The only document that cannot be changed this way is the person's birth certificate.

Many other European states insist that names come from a list of government approved, clearly gendered, names. The Registrar or administrative judge can refuse any name if they feel it does not 'match' the person making the application, or is not a recognised name. This is clearly problematic for non-binary persons as they will be compelled to have a formal name that is gendered. Also, trans people in general may be refused a 'non-matching' name (determined by someone else) which is nonetheless the most appropriate from a self-identification point of view.

Social Title and Pronouns

In the laws of the UK states (England and Wales; Scotland and Northern Ireland), there is no governance of pronouns; he, him, she, her—or personal titles; Mr, Ms, Mrs, Miss (or sir or madam). Only titles obtained through qualification, that is, Dr, Professor, Lord, Dame, and so on, are governed by law. Yet, pronouns and titles pervade our daily lives through social and employment practices, and interactions with law enforcement bodies or the courts. As a genderqueer in the UK puts it: "The trouble is, when someone is asking *us* for a title, they're basically asking if we're a guy or a girl. The answer is almost always neither" (2011).

The other complication is that whilst there is no legal governance of most titles, there is also no legal governance of potential gender-neutral titles, and thus institutional forms and computer programmes which require a title to be submitted rarely offer a gender-neutral option. Cassian, blogging in 2011 about one company's acknowledgement of the gender-neutral title *Mx*, enthused: "This is amazing because: [...] People who are or may be genderqueer but don't know about the title may see it when applying for deed poll documents, and feel accepted and recognised. The latter is a BIG DEAL. Non-binary people are basically invisible" (Cassian, 2011). Indeed, there is a petition on the UK Government and Parliament Petitions website seeking support for a requirement that government bodies should allow use of gender-neutral honorifics such as Mx (Petition, 2016). Whilst the intention is clearly good, the result might be formal recognition of gendered titles, and that would be very unsatisfactory.

As with titles, pronoun use is habitual and (in English, at least) grammatically gendered. The neutral pronoun *they* seems to have greater currency than *ze* or other neutral pronouns (see Nonbinary.org, 2016a), but its usage is far from universal.[7] However, this should not obscure the significant impact of repeated mis-gendering by pronoun or social title. A person with a non-binary gender identity cannot require a person to use appropriate pronouns, or titles—however, organisations or persons serious about respecting others will endeavour to use that person's preferred pronoun and title. For example, Christie Elan-Cane prefers the use of *per* and *perself* for per's pronouns. The members of the UK Parliament's Women and Equalities Committee managed to use the terms entirely successfully when Elan-Cane appeared before the Inquiry into Transgender Equality (Women and Equalities Committee 2016).

Formal Sex and Gender Designation

A person's legal sex is usually regarded as that designated on their birth certificate—it will refer to them as male or female. Essentially, it is a category resulting from a cursory examination by a midwife; their glance at the length of baby's primary sex organ will decide whether it is a penis or a clitoris. A midwife will only examine to see if a baby has a vagina if the primary sex organ is in the region of 2.4 cm, that is, too long to be one thing, too short to be another. Naturally occurring variations in biology are disregarded (Hines 2004; Roughgarden, 2004). The law's view of gender and sex is evolving; however, sex is still regarded as a physical 'fact,' and gender as a psychological experience (see Hines, 2004, p. 4, for discussion of why it is unfeasible to make this distinction).

Many nation and federal states now allow a person to obtain legal recognition of a preferred ('opposite') gender identity as if their birth sex (e.g. the *Gender Recognition Act*, 2004), but few allow full legal recognition of a non-binary gender identity as a legal sex. The Australian federal government allows people with medical evidence of gender reassignment (which need not be medical or surgical), intersex, or indeterminate sex, to have X as their gender marker on their passport, but as yet none of the Australian States allow that as a legal sex marker on birth registration documents.[8] New Zealand has allowed trans citizens, as well as those who are intersex, to obtain a passport with a preferred gender marker of X.[9] This is not, however, their legal sex, which is either that recorded at birth or after application for a change of birth registration—and this can only be 'male' or 'female' (Dept. Internal Affairs, n.d.-a) unless there is medical evidence that a person is of indeterminate sex or intersex (Dept. Internal Affairs, n.d.-b). Nepal makes 'O' (Other) passports available (Knight, 2015); and Pakistan also recognises a third gender apart from male and female in some circumstances (Maqbool, 2011). The only state to date which allows a person to choose to have X as their legal gender marker in all circumstances is Denmark (TransGender Europe, 2014).

In the UK, following earlier support for recognition of non-binary gender identities, an Early Day Motion was tabled for debate in the House of Commons 2016–2017 parliamentary session. Entitled *Legal recognition for people who do not associate with a particular gender*, it aimed to:

> address the issues faced by people whose identities are neither male nor female; [this House] believes that people are compromised and diminished as a result of inappropriate gender references on their personal identity information; […][and] notes that citizens of Australia and New Zealand are able to obtain a non-gender-specific X passport and that India, Nepal and Pakistan make provision for their citizens when neither M nor F are appropriate; further believes that similar provision is needed in the UK […] and therefore urges that […] non gender-specific X passports [are made] available […] to people who do not identify with a particular gender. (Lamb, 2016)

However, very few Early Day Motions will result in actual debate or legislative change.

Public Toilet Access for Non-binary People

The majority of public toilets in the UK are separated into male and female facilities, although increasingly non-segregated toilets can be found in universities, LGBT bars, and LGBT-friendly areas of cities (Ward, 2013), and at gender-inclusive events. However, as Kopas notes, echoing points made by Browne (2004), and Cavanagh (2010):

> Because gender-segregated public bathrooms allow for only two genders and hence set up the possibility of "failing" this gender test, public bathrooms are often sites of violence against gender non-conforming individuals, who may be the targets of interpersonal gender policing regardless of which gendered choice they make. (Kopas, 2012a, p. 9)

If toilets are marked male or female, it is unsurprising that non-binary people with non-conforming gender expression are accused of using the "wrong" bathroom (Cavanagh, 2010). Beliefs about segregation are clearly deep-rooted. Kopas notes that "The participants in my research were for the most part attached to the norm of gender separation, and even when participants' arguments were challenged on the grounds of being illogical or inconsistent, a strong resistance to removing gender segregation remained" (Kopas, 2012b).

UK law provides different rules regarding toilet provision, for employers and service providers, depending upon the building they occupy and what can reasonably be provided. A large office block or factory can clearly provide more toilet space than a small sandwich shop. Whatever the business, employers must always provide toilet facilities or allow reasonable access to other toilets outside of the workplace, for employees.

Local bye-laws may require places where people eat—such as restaurants—to provide toilets for patrons. For other services, the minimum is one toilet, which is also accessible to people with disabilities. After that, if it is feasible, provision should be made for a separate toilet for women from that used by men. However, there is no legal requirement for total separation. So long as one toilet is separate for women to use (and where possible, a separate one for men), all other toilets can be shared toilets. If there are toilets distinguished as men's and women's, there is no legal requirement that people only use one of the designated toilets.

The Equality Act (2010) requires that everyone, including trans people, is provided with the same access to facilities as any other person. If a person is presenting in their preferred gender identity, they must have the same access as others presenting in that gender identity—including access to changing rooms and the toilets. Managers and licensees of private premises have the right to decide who may enter the premises; though it is doubtful that they, rather than the provisions of the Equality Act, can determine who can access which toilet (Bishop, n.d.). The only time a person can be lawfully prevented access to a toilet is if a police officer (called by a manager, possibly) observes a person behaving in a way likely to cause a breach of the peace.

Recent years have seen a significant decline in the number of public toilets, and therefore an increase in the use of toilet facilities in shopping centres, pubs, and cafes (Department of Communities and Local Government, 2008). People with non-binary gender identities are invisible in government and policy documents on this issue. The decline of public toilets has had a disproportionate effect on women; older; disabled people, and carers of young children (Department of Communities and Local Government, 2008).

Prior to the Equality Act (2010), anti-discrimination law only concerned race, disabilities, and sex. Sex was about men and women, but there was recognition even then that the relative lack of women's public toilets was of real concern (Communities and Local Government Committee, 2008). The Equality Act (2010) advice provided for businesses who sell goods and services gives the following example:

Can a man just put on some lipstick and try to get into the ladies' toilet?

No. [...] a man who just puts on lipstick but does not wish to change his sex is not a transsexual person who is undergoing the process of changing his gender, nor is he likely to be thought to be transsexual, so he cannot rely on this protection. (British Chambers of Commerce and Government Equalities Office, 2010, p. 6)

A petition for gender-neutral public toilets exists in the archives for the 2010–2015 Conservative–Liberal Democrat UK coalition government (Archived Petition, 2010); it obtained just six signatures.

Relationship Recognition

Legal relationship recognition, comprising marriage and civil partnership, retains a binary-gendered framework. In 1866, a decision at the common law held that marriage as understood in Christendom is the voluntary union for life of one man and one woman, to the exclusion of all others.[10] In the requirements for marriage, most elements of that decision have long gone, with only 'one man and one woman' continuing to exist until the enactment of the Marriage (Same Sex Couples) Act (2013).

Legislative advances were made in the Gender Recognition Act (2004), which allowed trans people who obtained legal recognition to marry a person of the 'opposite' gender, rather than to marry in their birth assigned gender. However, those who had married in the former gender role were unable to get recognition of their preferred gender unless they ended their marriage. It was recognised that this could cause grave injustices especially for older couples, where employment-related survival pension benefits were often dependent upon the couple retaining a married status. This situation was ameliorated by the enactment of Civil Partnership Act in December 2004, which allowed same-sex couples to register a relationship akin to marriage, albeit not marriage in some small aspects. Combined with the provisions of the Gender Recognition Act (2004), and some clever footwork in the rules of Court, this allowed married trans people to end their marriage by annulment. The trans spouse would then receive a Gender Recognition Certificate, which enabled the couple to immediately contract a Civil Partnership, so protecting the survivor pension benefits of the (mostly non-trans) partner (former spouse).

In 2013, the UK government passed the Marriage (Same Sex Couples) Act, (2013). The Act allowed for equal marriage for same-sex couples (albeit without the religious elements, and not in Northern Ireland), but it did not at the same time allow 'opposite' sex couples to contract a civil partnership. The Act allows those couples in a civil partnership to convert the partnership to a marriage without having to go through a further ceremony. Importantly, for trans people seeking gender recognition, the Act allows for already-married trans people to obtain gender recognition without ending their marriage.

It can be seen that the legislative focus has so far been on relationship equality understood through a binary gender model. Non-binary persons at present must identify as either male or female in order to marry, a situation which is clearly unsatisfactory.

There is some prospect for change. *Ferguson and Others v. United Kingdom*, an application to the European Court of Human Rights case borne from the Equal Love Campaign (n.d.), was originally concerned with obtaining same-sex marriage (made redundant by the Marriage (Same Sex Couples) Act) and different-sex civil partnership. The application was declared inadmissible in 2015, but still has life in the domestic courts as *Steinfeld and Keidan* (Bowcott, 2016). Human rights cases such as these aim to broaden the application of Article 8 of the European Convention on Human Rights, which guarantees the right to respect for private and family life. If successful, either in the UK or the European Court of Human Rights, this would make gender-neutral formal relationships effective (cf. King, 2016).

Equality Act, 2010

The Equality Act, s. 4 (*Equality Act*, 2010), provides protection to people who have a *protected characteristic* being: age; disability; gender reassignment; marriage or civil partnership; pregnancy or maternity; race and ethnicity; religion or belief; sex; and sexual orientation. A person who has (or who is perceived to have) a protected characteristic is afforded protection from discrimination and harassment. This includes association with, or victimisation for supporting, a protected person. Public bodies are required to "give due regard to eliminating discrimination, harassment, victimisation [...]; advancing equality of opportunity; and fostering good relations, between persons with a protected characteristic and those who do not share it" (*Equality Act*, 2010, section 149).

In recent years, there has been a move towards making legislation sex or gender neutral (e.g. The Sexual Offences Act, 2003). However, the Equality Act (2010) retained the specification of sex, and the gender/sex binary in various *protected characteristics*. Sex is "a reference to a man or a woman" (Equality Act, 2010, section 11(a)), though the aim of the Act is to neutralise the impact of sex or gender. Sexual orientation is also binary: A person's sexual orientation towards persons of the same sex, persons of the 'opposite' sex, or of 'either' sex (section 12(1)). The characteristic of gender reassignment recognises people who are intending to undergo, are undergoing, or have undergone "a process (or part of a process) for the purpose of reassigning the person's sex by changing physiological or other attributes of sex" (section 7(1)), and according to the Act, this makes them a transsexual person.

There is no doubt that the Act was poorly conceived as regards gender identity concerns. The government used the language originally used by the Advocate General of the European Court of Justice, in the 1997 case of *P v. S & Cornwall County Council*.[11] In 2010, a consortium of trans support groups argued for the replacement of the narrow characteristic *gender reassignment* with *gender identity* in the proposed Equality Act, so providing protection to people with various gender identities which are different. This would include:

> Transsexual, transgender, or [other] gender variant identities, [...] would also protect children or adolescents without requiring them to choose to have gender reassignment [...] when their identities are still flexible and forming, be in line with the international human rights, equality and diversity statements, recommendations etc. of the UN, the Yogyakarta Principles, the Council of Europe, the EU, and others. (Press For Change, 2009, p. 2)

Their recommendation, which includes non-binary people in the reference to *gender variant identities*, was turned down, but just seven years later, the recommendations of the recent Inquiry of the House of Commons Women and Equalities Committee mirrored those words:

> The use of the terms "gender reassignment" and "transsexual" in the Act is outdated and misleading; and may not cover wider members of the trans

community. The protected characteristic in respect of trans people under the Equality Act should be amended to that of "gender identity" [...] bringing the language in the Act up to date, making it compliant with Council of Europe Resolution 2048; and make it significantly clearer that protection is afforded to anyone who might experience discrimination because of their gender identity.

Gender identities here need to be construed as including non-gendered identities to afford protection to people such as Christie Elan-Cane.

The explanatory notes to the Equality Act (2010) make it quite clear that 'gender reassignment' is to be considered a social process and not a medical process. As such, the Act protects anyone who "is intending to, is undergoing, or has undergone gender reassignment even if they have not had or do not intend to have any medical gender reassignment treatments" (Government Equalities Office, 2010, s.7, paras 41–43). However, what matters is that a person, at the very least, intends to permanently live in their preferred gender role. It is also clear that the Act is intended to exclude those who 'cross-dress' for reasons other than moving to live permanently in a gender role different to that assigned at birth. Similarly, in relation to the protected characteristic of sex:

A reference to a person who has a particular protected characteristic is a reference to a man or to a woman. (*Equality Act*, 2010, section 11)

A type of secondary protection from discrimination might be available to a person who has a non-binary gender identity in instances where:

A person (A) discriminates against another (B) if, because of a protected characteristic, A treats B less favourably than A treats or would treat others. (*Equality Act*, 2010, section 13(1))

This section does not *require* that (B) actually has the protected characteristic. So, if a person is wrongly perceived to be intending to undergo gender reassignment, or to be gay or lesbian or bisexual, and treated less favourably because of that, this would constitute unlawful discrimination on the grounds of gender reassignment or sexual orientation under the Act 2010.

Similarly, harassment occurs where a person engages in unwanted conduct "related to a relevant protected characteristic" (*Equality Act*, 2010, section 26). The Code of Practice makes it clear that harassment is possible where there is any connection with a protected characteristic, whether or not the person themselves has that characteristic. If a person with a non-binary gender identity is harassed because they are wrongly assumed to have a protected characteristic such as gender reassignment or being gay or lesbian or bisexual, they can obtain protection under the Act (see Great Britain and Equality and Human Rights Commission, 2011, paragraphs 7.10 and 7.11, for further discussion).

Aileen McColgan of Matrix Chambers suggests, when discussing cross dressing, that there may be cases in which discrimination because of a person's wearing 'inappropriate clothing' for their recorded birth sex could constitute sex discrimination. However, "the domestic courts have remained very reluctant to interfere with employers' rights to impose 'gender appropriate' clothing and appearance rules" (McColgan, 2014, paragraph 4).

Gender Recognition

In addition to this gender binary focus, UK law has an emphasis on official recognition or approval before a change in gender becomes recognised in law. The Gender Recognition Act requires evidence of a person having been diagnosed with Gender Dysphoria. (*Gender Recognition Act*, 2004, section 1). The diagnosis of gender identity disorder has now been superseded by a diagnosis of gender dysphoria, which is far wider in its conception as: "A marked incongruence between one's experienced/expressed gender and assigned gender" (APA, para 302.85). The likely forthcoming version of the ICD-11 also looks set to 'declassify' Gender Dysphoria, rename it Gender Incongruence, and position Gender Incongruence in a non-mental health chapter (currently, a chapter likely entitled *Conditions related to sexual health*; World Health Organization, 2016).

Ireland, on the other hand, has followed the example of Argentina and Denmark, and the intended direction of other European countries

(O'Toole, 2015) in allowing citizens to apply for a Gender Recognition on the basis of self-declaration (*Gender Recognition Act*, 2015; Transgender Equality Network Ireland, n.d.). Although the Irish Gender Recognition Act does not have a provision for self-definition as having a third gender or no gender, self-definition is likely to lead to these options having to be considered. If the defining characteristic of gender is self-perception, then there is no logical reason for self-perception to be restricted to the male/female binary. In contrast, however, a system in which authority rests outside the hands of the persons requiring recognition of their gender seems more likely to be conservative when faced with new gender possibilities.

Gender Identity Protection in Scottish Law

UK law is binary-focussed when it addresses questions of gender identity. There is one exception; the Offences (Aggravation by Prejudice) (Scotland) Act (2009), which provides a statutory aggravation for offences where the accused has evinced malice or ill will relating to sexual orientation or transgender identity. Transgender identity is defined as:

(a) transvestism, transsexualism, intersexuality, or having, by virtue of the Gender Recognition Act (2004) (c.7), changed gender, or;
(b) any other gender identity that is not standard male or female gender identity (*Offences (Aggravation by Prejudice) (Scotland) Act*, 2009 section 2(8)(a) and (b)).

The Yogyakarta Principles

The Yogyakarta Principles (International Commission of Jurists and International Service for Human Rights, 2007), whilst not having been adopted as law by any national, federal, or supra-national body; and having no binding effect in international human rights law; have however been acknowledged as influential. Unsurprisingly, given the pedigree of the human rights experts who authorised the principles, the definition of gender identity in the *Principles* is exemplary. Gender identity is:

To refer to each person's deeply felt internal and individual experience of gender, which may or may not correspond with the sex assigned at birth, including the personal sense of the body (which may involve, if freely chosen, modification of bodily appearance or function by medical, surgical or other means) and other expressions of gender, including dress, speech and mannerisms. (International Commission of Jurists and International Service for Human Rights, 2007, Preamble)

Given the non-binding status of the *Principles,* it might be thought that they are richer in potential than effectiveness, and reservations have been expressed by Dreyfus (2012) and Waites (2009). However, O'Flaherty and Fisher (2008) argue that the *Principles,* read in conjunction with General Comments of the United Nations human rights treaties bodies on States' obligations to undertake effective programmes of education and public awareness about human rights, and general duty to enable people to benefit from their entitlements, ought to have significant impact.

Following the Yogyakarta Principles, it is generally considered clear that international human rights law now contains the general principle that that all persons, regardless of sexual orientation or gender identity, are entitled to the full enjoyment of all human rights. Following the *Recommendation CM/Rec(2010)5 of the European Council Committee of Ministers on measures to combat discrimination on grounds of sexual orientation or gender identity,* in 2011, the European Union amended the Qualification Directive 2004/83/EC[12] to include explicit reference to gender identity; Article 10(1)(d) of the Directive now reads: "Gender related aspects, including gender identity, shall be given due consideration for the purposes of determining membership of a particular social group or identifying a characteristic of such a group."

According to Tsourdi, this means the Directive also entails an obligation for decision-makers to give consideration to gender-related aspects, including gender identity—reflected by the use of "shall" instead of "might." Even with this strengthened wording, however, and the inclusion of gender identity, it does not unambiguously include intersex individuals, although the Directive does recognise in Article 9(2) that gender-specific acts and child-specific acts fall within the concept of persecution and both of these references can be relevant in cases of persecution of intersex people (2013).

Future Directions

The recently published report on Transgender Equality by the Women and Equalities Committee makes a number of positive observations and significant recommendations, including the following. These recommendations are striking, both individually and in their totality:

> 5. The Government must look into the need to create a legal category for those people with a gender identity outside that which is binary and the full implications of this.

> 7. Within the current Parliament, the Government must bring forward proposals to update the Gender Recognition Act, in line with the principles of gender self-declaration that have been developed in other jurisdictions. In place of the present medicalised, quasi-judicial application process, an administrative process must be developed, centred on the wishes of the individual applicant, rather than on intensive analysis by doctors and lawyers.

> 13. We recommend that provision should be made to allow 16- and 17-year-olds, with appropriate support, to apply for gender recognition, on the basis of self-declaration.

> 17. The inclusion of "gender reassignment" as a protected characteristic in the Equality Act (2010) was a huge step forward and has clearly improved the position of trans people. However, it is clear to us that the use of the terms "gender reassignment" and "transsexual" in the Act is outdated and misleading; and may not cover wider members of the trans community.

> 18. The protected characteristic in respect of trans people under the Equality Act should be amended to that of "gender identity". This would improve the law by bringing the language in the Act up to date, making it compliant with Council of Europe Resolution 2048; and make it significantly clearer that protection is afforded to anyone who might experience discrimination because of their gender identity.

56. The UK must follow Australia's lead in introducing an option to record gender as "X" on a passport. If Australia is able to implement such a policy there is no reason why the UK cannot do the same. In the longer term, consideration should be given to the removal of gender from passports.

57. The Government should be moving towards "non-gendering" official records as a general principle and only recording gender where it is a relevant piece of information. Where information on gender is required for monitoring purposes, it should be recorded separately from individuals' personal records and only subject to the consent of those concerned. (Women and Equalities Committee, 2015, pp. 79–87)

If even a fraction of the recommendations of the Committee are put into effect, these will make a significant improvement to the legal recognition of people with non-binary gender identities.

Conclusions

Law engages as much with the lives of people with non-binary gender identities, as it does with others, but being non-binary repeatedly highlights law's patriarchal heteronormative history whilst frequently frustrating law's purpose. Law cannot recognise a world containing a plurality of gender identities, because it was constructed to uphold the point of difference contained in a binary-gendered system.

However, the law is not static, and advances are being made through the work of theorists and activists. There is currently inadequate recognition of, and protection for, people with non-binary gender identities, but it is not without hope that change will appear in the near future. It is clear that those drafting the Equality Act (2010) (albeit within a restricted concept formed in mid-1990s employment law) intended the law to be far reaching in its protection of people who were gender diverse. As it stands however, people with non-binary gender identities are not bringing discrimination and/or equality cases to court—quite reasonably when legal aid is not available to most, and legal support which will be needed to bring a successful challenge is expensive and beyond the reach of people who have struggled to get and keep the job they have. The alternative is probably not to seek legislative change head on, but rather to seek regulatory change of minor parts of the Act. Simply changing gender reassignment to gender identity in the Act will resolve the major part of the problem, and provide clear and extensive protection.

Legislation is best when it works by stealth—not through the courts. And just as minor changes to the Equality Act (2010) would bring huge advances, minor changes to the Gender Recognition Act (2004) would bring great change. By looking to the experience of other nations, it is clear that the systems of self-identification favoured in other jurisdictions are working—and that the sky has not fallen down.

Understanding that gender is like race—nothing more than a system developed to give power to some, and to keep other powerless, would be a start. But that is not in itself enough. We also have to acknowledge that for most, having some sort of gender identity, or not having a gender identity at all, is a keenly felt essential part of their autonomous, independent self. To acknowledge that universality in law without being prescriptive would enhance the well-being of many—without damaging anyone else's sense of self. Comprehending the plurality of gender identities is not an especially novel idea; indeed, the jurists, lawyers, and activists behind the Yogyakarta Principles got to grips with it ten years ago (2007). This flourishing of a more inclusive conception of gender has borne fruit in the recognition of this plurality in the recent report of the Parliamentary Women and Equalities Committee whose recommendations, if given effect, should significantly impact for the better lives of people in the UK with non-binary gender identities.

Notes

1. With grateful thanks to Nathan Gale and Tony Ward for their comments and suggestions in an unreasonably short timeframe.
2. There are political connotations to some of these terms, especially 'genderqueer' that 'non-binary' may obscure (Nonbinary.org, 2016b).
3. Transsexual is a medical category used to refer to people who seek out gender reassignment treatments and/or surgery to enable them to live in a preferred gender role different to that ascribed at birth.

4. Transgender is becoming the term of choice amongst Governmental bodies, as it is an inclusive term, which includes those people referred to as transsexual and those people who live in a preferred gender role that is different to that ascribed at birth with limited or without medical intervention.

5. See the 'transsexual cases' at the European Court of Human Rights such as Rees v United Kingdom [1987] 9 EHRR 56., Cossey v United Kingdom [1991] 13 EHRR 622., and Sheffield and Horsham v United Kingdom [1999] 27 EHRR 163.

6. Elan-Cane requests use of the terms *per* and *perself* rather than gendered pronouns.

7. For a facetious take on everyday pronoun interactions, see Beyondthebinary (2016).

8. See sex and gender diverse passport applicants at https://www.passports.gov.au/passportsexplained/theapplicationprocess/eligibilityoverview/Pages/changeofsexdoborpob.aspx.

9. See information about changing sex/gender identity at https://www.passports.govt.nz/Transgender-applicants, and Denmark: X in Passports and New Trans Law Works at http://tgeu.org/denmark-x-in-passports-and-new-trans-law-work/.

10. Penzance, LJ, in Hyde v. Hyde and Woodmansee. [L.R.] 1 P. & D. 130.

11. P v. S and Cornwall County Council, Case C-13/94, [1996] IRLR 347.

12. The Qualification Directive 2004/83/EC of 29 April 2004 sets up the Common European Asylum System (CEAS).

References

Archived Petition: Gender Neutral Public Toilets. (2010). *Petitions—UK Government and Parliament.* Retrieved January 29, 2016, from https://petition.parliament.uk/archived/petitions/75908

Bishop, J.-A. (n.d.). *The Toilet Issue—Which Toilet should Trans* People Use?* Retrieved January 29, 2016, from http://www.antheamakepeace.co.uk/toiletissue.pdf

Bornstein, K. (1994). *Gender Outlaw: On Men, Women and the Rest of Us.* New York: Taylor & Francis.

British Chambers of Commerce, Government Equalities Office. (2010). *Equality Act 2010: What Do I Need to Know? A Summary Guide for Businesses*

Who Sell Goods and Services. Retrieved January 29, 2016, from https://www.gov.uk/government/uploads/system/uploads/attachment_data/file/85009/business-summary.pdf

Browne, K. (2004). Genderism and the Bathroom Problem: (Re)materialising Sexed Sites, (Re)creating Sexed Bodies. *Gender, Place & Culture, 11*, 331–346.

Cavanagh, S. L. (2010). *Queering Bathrooms: Gender, Sexuality and the Hygienic Imagination*. Toronto: University of Toronto Press.

Civil Partnership Act. (2004).

Coleman, E., Bockting, W., Botzer, M., Cohen-Kettenis, P., Decuypere, P., Feldman, G., et al. (2012). Standards of Care for the Health of Transsexual, Transgender, and Gender-Nonconforming People, Version 7. *International Journal of Transgenderism, 13*(4), 165–232.

Communities and Local Government Committee. (2008). *The Provision of Public Toilets (House of Commons No. HC 636), Twelfth Report of Session 2007–2008*. London: The Stationary Office.

Department for Communities and Local Government. (2008). *Improving Public Access to Better Quality Toilets. A Strategic Guide*. London: Department for Communities and Local Government.

Department of Internal Affairs. (n.d.-a). *General Information Regarding Declarations of Family Court as to Sex to be Shown on Birth Certificates*. Wellington, New Zealand: Dept. of Internal Affairs. Retrieved February 2, 2016, from https://www.dia.govt.nz/diawebsite.nsf/Files/GeninfoDeclaratio nsofFamilyCourt/$file/GeninfoDeclarationsofFamilyCourt.pdf

Department of Internal Affairs. (n.d.-b). *Citizenship Office Policy for Transgender and Intersex Applicants*. Wellington, New Zealand: Dept. of Internal Affairs. Retrieved February 2, 2016, from https://www.dia.govt.nz/diawebsite.nsf/Files/Citpol15 Transgenderandintersexcitapp/$file/Citpol15Transgenderandintersexcitapp.pdf

Dreyfus, T. (2012). The "Half-Invention" of Gender Identity in International Human Rights Law: From Cedaw to the Yogyakarta Principles. *Australian Feminist Law Journal, 37*, 33–50.

Elan-Cane, C. (2011) Non-Gendered: Fighting for Legal and Social Recognition Outside the Gendered Societal Structure. *Christie Elan-Cane Live Journal Profile*. Retrieved February 2, 2016, from http://elancane.livejournal.com/2011/02/02/

Equality Act. (2010).

Equality and Human Rights Commission. (2011). *Employment: Statutory Code of Practice*. London: EHRC.

Fraser, L. (2015). Gender Dysphoria: Definition and Evolution Through the Years. In C. Trombetta, G. Liguori, & M. Bertolotto (Eds.), *Management of Gender Dysphoria: A Multidisciplinary Approach* (pp. 19–32). Milan: Springer-Verlag Italia.

Gender Recognition Act. (2004).

Gender Recognition Act. (2015).

Government Equalities Office. (2010). *Equality Act 2010 Explanatory Notes*. Retrieved February 5, 2016, from http://www.legislation.gov.uk/ukpga/2010/15/notes

Hines, M. (2004). *Brain Gender*. Oxford: Oxford University Press.

International Commission of Jurists, International Service for Human Rights. (2007). *The Yogyakarta Principles: Principles on the Application of International Human Rights Law in Relation to Sexual Orientation and Gender Identity*. Geneva: International Commission of Jurists.

Jeffreys, S. (2015). *Written Evidence to the House of Commons Women and Equalities Committee Inquiry into Transgender Equality*. Retrieved January 12, 2016, from http://data.parliament.uk/writtenevidence/committeeevidence.svc/evidencedocument/women-and-equalities-committee/transgender-equality/written/19512.html

King, K. (2016). *I Went to Watch the Civil Partnerships Case at the High Court and Even the Judge Didn't Understand It*. Legal Cheek. Retrieved January 29, 2016, from http://www.legalcheek.com/2016/01/i-went-to-watch-the-civil-partnerships-case-at-the-high-court-and-even-the-judge-didnt-understand-it/

Knight, K. (2015). *Nepal's Third Gender Passport Blazes Trails*. Human Rights Watch. Retrieved January 29, 2016, from https://www.hrw.org/news/2015/10/26/nepals-third-gender-passport-blazes-trails

Kopas, M. (2012a). *The Illogic of Separation: Examining Arguments About Gender-Neutral Public Bathrooms*. Master's Thesis (MA Sociology). University of Washington, Washington, DC.

Kopas, M. (2012b). *Research On/For Whom? Lessons Learned From Studying Public Bathrooms*. Retrieved from http://mkopas.net/files/Kopas_AGREAA-Trans-Studies_2012_text.pdf

Lamb, N. (2016). *Early Day Motion 11—Legal Recognition for People Who Do Not Associate with a Particular Gender*. Retrieved August 25, 2016, from https://www.parliament.uk/edm/2016-17/11

Maqbool, A. (2011). *Pakistan Allows Transsexuals to Have Own Gender Category*. Retrieved January 29, 2016, from http://www.bbc.co.uk/news/world-south-asia-13192077

Marriage (Same Sex Couples) Act. (2013).

Nonbinary.org. (2016a). *Pronouns.* Retrieved January 31, 2016, from http://nonbinary.org/wiki/Pronouns#Per

Nonbinary.org. (2016b). *Genderqueer.* Nonbinary.org. Retrieved January 28, 2016, from http://nonbinary.org/wiki/Genderqueer

O'Flaherty, M., & Fisher, J. (2008). Sexual Orientation, Gender Identity and International Human Rights Law: Contextualising the Yogyakarta Principles. *Human Rights Law Review, 8,* 207–248.

O'Toole, M. (2015). 6 Reasons Why the UK's Gender Laws Are Failing Transgender People. *PinkNews.* Retrieved January 28, 2016, from http://www.pinknews.co.uk/2015/10/15/6-reasons-why-the-uks-gender-laws-are-failing-transgender-people/

Offences (Aggravation by Prejudice) (Scotland) Act. (2009).

Petition: Require Government Bodies to Allow Use of Gender-Neutral Honorifics e.g. "Mx". (2016). *Petitions—UK Government and Parliament.* Retrieved January 29, 2016, from https://petition.parliament.uk/petitions/119655

Press For Change. (2009). *The Equality Bill 2009: PFC's Proposed Amendments: A Short Guide.* London: Press For Change.

Raymond, J. G. (1979). *The Transsexual Empire: The Making of the She-Male.* Boston, MA: Beacon Press.

Roughgarden, J. (2004). *Evolution's Rainbow: Diversity, Gender and Sexuality in Nature and People.* Berkeley: University of California Press.

Self, W., & Gamble, D. (2000). *Perfidious Man.* London: Viking.

Stone, S. (1992). The Empire Strikes Back: A Posttranssexual Manifesto. *Camera Obscura: Feminism, Culture, and Media. Studies, 10*(229), 150–176.

Stryker, S. (1994). My Words to Victor Frankenstein Above the Village of Chamounix: Performing Transgender Rage. *GLQ: A Journal of Lesbian and Gay Studies, 1*(3), 237–254.

Stryker, S., & Whittle, S. (Eds.). (2006). *The Transgender Studies Reader.* New York: Taylor & Francis.

The Yogyakarta Principles. (2007). *The Yogyakarta Principles on the Application of International Human Rights Law in Relation to Sexual Orientation and Gender Identity.* Retrieved February 5, 2016, from http://www.yogyakartaprinciples.org/principles_en.pdf

Transgender Equality Network Ireland. (n.d.). *Legal Gender Recognition in Ireland: Gender Recognition: TENI.* Retrieved January 29, 2016, from http://www.teni.ie/page.aspx?contentid=586

Transgender Europe. (2014). *Denmark: X in Passports and New Trans Law Works*. Retrieved February 2, 2016, from http://tgeu.org/denmark-x-in-passports-and-new-trans-law-work/

Tsourdi, E. (Lilian). (2013). Sexual Orientation and Gender Identity: Developments in EU Law. *Forced Migration Review, 42*, 20–21.

Waites, M. (2009). Critique of "Sexual Orientation" and "Gender Identity" in Human Rights Discourse: Global Queer Politics Beyond the Yogyakarta Principles. *Contemporary Politics, 15*, 137–156.

Williams, W. L. (1988). *The Spirit and the Flesh, Sexual Diversity. In American Indian Culture*. Boston, MA: Beacon Press.

Women and Equalities Committee. (2015). *Transgender Equality (No. First Report of Session 2015–16)*. London: House of Commons.

World Health Organization. (2016). *ICD-11 Beta Draft—Joint Linearization for Mortality and Morbidity Statistics*. World Health Organization. Retrieved August 26, 2016, from http://apps.who.int/classifications/icd11/browse/l-m/en#/http%3a%2f%2fid.who.int%2ficd%2fentity%2f90875286

Zagria. (2013). *Louis Gradon Sullivan (1951–1991) Pioneer FTM Activist. A Gender Variance Who's Who*. Retrieved February 2, 2016, from http://zagria.blogspot.ca/2008/07/louis-gradon-sullivan-1951-1991-pioneer.html#.VrAw9fmLRVz

Part II

Minds

6

Psychotherapy

Meg-John Barker and Alex Iantaffi

Introduction

In this chapter, we provide an overview of psychotherapeutic and coun-selling practice with non-binary clients. After a brief introduction to non-binary clients and the general mental health of this client group, we explore the ways in which the major psychotherapeutic approaches (humanistic, psychodynamic, and cognitive-behavioural) conceptualise gender identity and expression, and the potential tensions and possibili-ties of these conceptualisations in relation to non-binary experience. We also offer ideas and practices from the existential and systemic therapeutic approaches, which often utilise less binary conceptualisations of gender.

M.-J. Barker (✉)
The Open University, Milton Keynes, Buckinghamshire, UK

A. Iantaffi
University of Minnesota, Minneapolis, MN, USA

© The Author(s) 2017
C. Richards et al. (eds.), *Genderqueer and Non-Binary Genders*, Critical and Applied
Approaches in Sexuality, Gender and Identity, DOI 10.1057/978-1-137-51053-2_6

Following this, we cover the content and process of therapy and counselling with non-binary people in more depth, highlighting the importance of not assuming any link between a client's non-binary gender and their presenting issues. However, we argue that it still behoves the practitioner to have enough understanding of non-binary gender to address, and engage with, non-binary clients in an appropriate, welcoming, and supportive manner which does not pathologise their gender. We explore common issues which non-binary people bring to therapy which *are* related to their gender, and how practitioners might work with such issues, while being mindful of the diversity of non-binary people and experiences. We draw out key ethical and practical issues when working with non-binary clients as a binary—or non-binary—practitioner, for example, in relation to therapist self-disclosure, client monitoring and assessment, and the use of client name and pronouns in session. Alternatives to conventional therapy, such as community support, self-care, and engagement with online resources, are also mentioned.

We conclude the chapter with a bullet point summary of best practice when working with non-binary clients.

Non-binary Clients

As mentioned in the introduction to this book, when discussing non-binary clients, we are referring to the small proportion of people who explicitly identify as non-binary, genderqueer, or one of the many other terms that fall under these umbrellas, and we are also talking about the far larger proportion of people who experience and express themselves in ways that fall between, or outside of, the binary of male and female.

As practitioners, we need to be open to all possibilities of identification, expression, and experience, rather than making assumptions about a particular client. Early on it may well be useful to ascertain where each individual client currently falls on a spectrum from identity to experience, as well as determining what their particular gender identity/experience is, and whether or not they are embedded within wider communities (and, if so, which). Other identities also need to be considered, especially racial or cultural identities, which might deeply impact a client's sense of self in relation to gender (see Iantaffi & Barker, 2017). Similarly, as we will discuss in more depth later, there will likely be ongoing dialogue in relation to how central gender is to the person's life and presenting issues, and how keen they are to engage with any formal gender services.

Non-binary People and Mental Health

There has been limited research so far on the mental health of non-binary people. However, what evidence there is strongly suggests that those who identify as non-binary have worse mental health than the general population, and possibly even than binary trans people (see Barker & Richards, 2015). For example, McNeil, Bailey, Ellis, Morton, and Regan (2012) found that those who identify as non-binary and/or express themselves in ways that explicitly challenge binary gender face similarly high levels of mental health difficulties to those of trans people more generally. Harrison, Grant and Herman (2012) found that over 40% of non-binary people had attempted suicide at some point, a third had experienced physical assault, and a sixth sexual assault based on their gender: experiences which we know are strongly related to psychological distress. These rates were even higher than for trans men and women (see the next two chapters for more relating to psychology and psychiatry).

Regarding the likely explanations for these disturbing findings, we might look to the wider literatures on trans and on bisexuality. Research on trans issues generally links high levels of distress and high suicide rates to the common experience of explicit and implicit transphobia, and to living in a cisgenderist world which assumes that people will remain in the gender that they were assigned at birth (Lenihan, Kainth & Dundas, 2015; Murjan & Bouman, 2015). Trans people also often feel pressure to conform to cisgenderist, binary views of gender in order to "fit in" and be seen as "legitimate" (Iantaffi & Bockting, 2011). Non-binary people are likely to share such experiences with binary trans people.

While cisgender bisexual people do not share the gender experiences of binary and non-binary trans people, they do share the experience of falling outside of heteronormative binary understandings of sexuality and gender (see Stewart, this volume; Barker & Scheele, 2016).

Heteronormativity and monosexuality are based upon the linked assumptions that sexuality is binary (straight or gay) and gender is binary (male or female). Bisexual people trouble the former, and non-binary people trouble the latter. The evidence is overwhelming that bisexual people in heteronormative and homonormative cultures experience worse mental health than either heterosexual or lesbian/gay people, probably due to the biphobia, erasure, and invisibility they experience for falling outside of the sexuality binary (Barker, Richards, Jones, Bowes-Catton, & Plowman 2012; Barker, 2015a). It is likely that this is similarly true for non-binary people: Falling outside the gender binary means that they experience erasure and invisibility (people rarely recognising or validating their gender), and discrimination on the basis of not fitting either side of the binary (particularly if they are visibly non-binary in any way).

Barker and Richards (2015) point to a further intriguingly possible reason for the particularly high levels of psychological distress amongst non-binary people. Psychological research has generally found that priming people to foreground their gender causes them to have lower confidence, self-esteem, and ability on gender-stereotyped tasks which do not match that gender. For example, if women are encouraged to consider gender stereotypes around maths, or even just to tick a gender box prior to being tested, they tend to perform worse on maths problems and demonstrate lower self-worth in this area (see Fine, 2010 for an overview of such research). Of course we live in a world where everyone is constantly primed for binary genders (male/female toilet doors, being called sir/madam, lining up as boys and girls in school, unnecessarily gendered products, etc.) It seems likely that this may have a similarly adverse impact on non-binary people's emotions, self-worth, and capabilities.

There is a further important and intriguing finding in relation to non-binary mental health, and that is that whilst non-binary identity seems related to poorer mental health, research dating back decades suggests that non-binary experience can actually be linked to better mental health, compared to binary experience of gender. Bem's studies from the 1970s to the 1990s consistently found that androgyny (by which she meant scoring highly on measures of both masculinity and femininity) was related to greater flexibility and psychological healthiness (e.g. Bem, 1995; Bem & Lenney, 1976).

We have worked with people on a spectrum from those who identify with a specific non-binary label and have a clear therapeutic aim in relation to that (such as coming out; negotiating a binary world as a non-binary person; or accessing gender transition services), through to those who see themselves as trans but feel that they only want to engage with some elements of 'conventional' binary gender transition (see Richards et al., 2015); through to those who have no non-binary or trans identities, but present with some sense of not experiencing themselves as male or female; to those who make no mention of gender, but for whom it emerges their emotional or relational issues are related to some level of discomfort or mis-fitting with their birth-assigned gender (e.g. in relation to their body, relationships, sexual experience, and/or emotional experience).

Such a spectrum ironically challenges any clear binary between non-binary and binary people. At which point on the spectrum would we draw that line? It also challenges the border between trans and cisgender people, given that we could say that none of these people have remained in the gender that they were assigned at birth, but not all would regard themselves—or be regarded as—trans. Indeed, Titman (2014) reports that only around a third of non-binary people confidently identify as trans, despite their experience of gender being encompassed by the term. Non-binary gender identities seem to be located in a more liminal space, where easy dichotomies and distinctions between trans and cis people are challenged and redefined.

Another important point to mention here is that there is also a great deal of diversity in how much clients engage with non-binary community or activism (see Barker & Bergman, this volume), and this certainly influences their identities and experiences. For example, a client who is very engaged with non-binary, trans, and/or queer communities may well have spent some time determining exactly which non-binary label best captures their gender experience (e.g. are they gender neutral; or experiencing of 'both' genders; or gender fluid; or political about challenging the binary gender system). They may also have a clear idea regarding their names, pronouns, and any bodily changes they wish to make. Somebody who is not engaged with communities may have far less sense of these possibilities, and might even [incorrectly] perceive some of their struggles as pathological.

Clearly, it is important to be mindful that those who identify and/ or express their gender in non-binary ways are at very high risk when it comes to mental health difficulties, self-harm, and suicide (Harrison, Grant, & Herman, 2012; McNeil, Bailey, Ellis, Morton, & Regan, 2012). However, it is also important to emphasise that non-binary experience per se has no relation to psychopathology—probably quite the opposite (Barker & Richards, 2013)—and that, as with LGBT people more generally, non-binary people are generally highly resilient due to what they have to overcome on a daily basis (Nodin, Peel, Tyler, & Rivers, 2015). The distress and struggles that non-binary people do face are likely to be largely due to transphobia and the minority/marginalisation stress of living in an often coercively binary world in which binary gender divisions are enforced through everything from everyday interactions to governmental policies and societal structures (e.g. passports and monitoring forms—see Clucas and Whittle this volume; Iantaffi & Bockting, 2011).

Therefore, perhaps *the* key issue that most non-binary clients face, whether or not they want to address it in therapy, is how best to navigate an overwhelmingly binary world as a non-binary person. We will come back to this, and other related issues, shortly.

Psychotherapeutic Modalities

A vital point to make when considering psychotherapy and counselling for non-binary clients is that all of the major therapeutic approaches have either an implicit, or often explicit, binary understanding of gender. This means that most practitioners are likely to assume that their clients will be either male or female, and that most will be at best confused—and at worst dismissive—when confronted with a non-binary client.

Furthermore, very few counselling or psychotherapy trainings include considerations of gender in any depth at all. Like race, sexuality, class, and other social structures, many trainers, supervisors, and the like do not recognise the vital role of gender in mental health, and focus more on the individual experience than on shared experiences of oppression or marginalisation (Barker, 2010). Given the lack of attention paid to gender, it is unsurprising that very few training courses make any mention of trans issues at all, and therefore coverage of non-binary genders is vanishingly rare (Davies & Barker, 2015).

Indeed, when we set up an online group for non-binary therapists, we found that they shared markedly similar experiences of raising the topics of gender, trans, and non-binary on their training courses. Most found that they—as non-binary people—had to educate their teachers and supervisors on these matters, and that they were met with confusion and occasionally pathologisation and stigmatisation. Certainly, courses and placements were not set up with them in mind, with many of them having to negotiate difficulties with placements which were looking purely for 'male' or 'female' therapists. Virtually all found that they became the lone voice on their courses on matters of gender (and often other sociocultural matters too) given the tendency of tutors and peers to see psychological distress only on an individual level. This is despite the known disparities between men and women; heterosexual and gay/bisexual people; cisgender and trans people; and white and black and minority ethnic (BME) people, when it comes to mental health diagnoses and psychological distress—and the known links between these aspects and experiences of marginalisation, discrimination, and the like (Barker, 2010).

Turning to specific psychotherapies, the dominant approaches are generally recognised as being psychodynamic, cognitive-behavioural, and humanistic (Barker, Vossler, & Langdridge, 2010), with many training courses offering some form of integrative, eclectic, or pluralistic combination of these approaches. All of these approaches explicitly or implicitly assume that gender is binary.

Psychodynamic approaches are probably the most explicit in their binary conceptualisations of gender. Obviously, the Freudian psychoanalysis that much psychodynamic therapy is grounded on is entirely binary and has clear notions about the normal and healthy trajectory that a man, and a woman, should take in terms of their psychological and sexual development. It would therefore seem difficult for a Freudian analyst to encounter a non-binary person without pathologising them. Similarly, several of the branches of psychoanalysis which followed Freud are inherently binary in their assumptions; for example, Jungian archetypes tend to be masculine or feminine, object relations theories and attachment theories tend to assume binary gender parents and gender roles, and Erikson's developmental stages assume a heteronormative gendered life trajectory. Whilst more recent psychoanalysts such as Lacan and Irigary, as well as those who draw on them such as Butler, have proposed far more sophisticated and nuanced understandings of gender—which more easily encompass non-binary experience—few counselling and psychotherapy courses teach the work of these thinkers. Practitioners may find it useful to familiarise themselves with the basics of these theories (see Stewart, this volume) and to draw upon them with clients. For example, Butler's idea that *all* gender is performative can be helpful to share with non-binary clients to reassure them that their experience is no less 'real' than that of people with binary genders.

Cognitive-behavioural therapy (CBT) is perhaps less obviously binary in its approach, and gender is far less central to its theories of human experience. However, CBT generally draws to a great extent on mainstream psychological research which is highly binary in its understandings of gender, and has generally ignored or pathologised trans experience until recent years. Psychological understandings of gender tend to be framed in terms of gender *difference*, categorising people as male and female and searching for differences between them. Thus, it assumes that gender categories are (a) binary and (b) meaningful (see Richards, this volume, for a more detailed consideration). In particular, the mainstream cognitive psychological theories of gender development tend to build on the likes of Kohlberg who operate entirely within a binary system, theorising how girls and boys take on board gender roles and come to a consistent gender identity. Bem's gender theories offer an alternative to this understanding which fits within mainstream psychology but opens up space for non-binary experiences. For example, she researched androgyny as psychologically healthy in its flexibility, and saw gender schemas as learnt rather than innate. However, we have rarely heard of Bem being taught on CBT trainings. This is a shame as it may well be empowering for non-binary clients to hear about these ideas in order to validate their often invalidated experience.

Finally, humanistic therapies are perhaps the least obviously binary of the three main approaches with more emphasis in early writings on the experience of being—or becoming—a person than specifically a man or a woman. However, like Kohlberg's theories, Maslow's hierarchy of needs has been criticised for gender bias in terms of which values it prioritises, and certainly, neither Rogers nor Maslow incorporates any explicit possibility for non-binary gender into their writings. However, humanistic ideas, such as conditions of worth, potentially offer a valuable way of understanding how everyone—non-binary people included—comes to experience stereotypical gender norms as restrictive, and there is potential in the core condition of unconditional positive regard to affirm the lived experience of non-binary clients in a world which often does the opposite. Perhaps the most valuable practice that we have found with clients who are exploring their non-binary gender is to provide them with a space in which to do this which is entirely open and affirming of all possible gender experiences and all possible options which they might wish to pursue.

Moving away from the dominant approaches to psychotherapy, other approaches have much to offer here, notably the existential and systemic therapeutic approaches which are generally grounded in less binary conceptualisations of gender.

Existential psychotherapy generally regards our gender as something that we *become* rather than something that we fundamentally *are*, and therefore implicitly includes the possibility of multiple gender identities and experiences. The writings of Simone de Beauvoir in particular are useful when working with non-binary clients given that she regards rigid binary gender roles as restrictive and highly linked to human suffering (see Barker, 2011). A key tension which many non-binary clients grapple with is that between the following two possibilities:

* Identifying and expressing themselves in ways which feel more authentic, but which leave them more open to being stigmatised and discriminated against by others, and
* Adhering to more conventional gender expression, but feeling a constant painful sense of not being themselves.

Clients have described this sense of inauthenticity as a weight that becomes heavier day on day. They also speak of the painful sense of being scrutinised that they can experience when they are expressing themselves in more authentic ways.

As Richards (2011, 2017) has pointed out, existential therapy has much to offer clients struggling with such tensions given its focus on authenticity, choice, the anxiety of uncertainty, and the leap to faith. It is vital here not to leap ahead of the client but to remain with their lived experience of uncertainty. We have found it useful, for example, to explore client's embodied sense when imagining each possible choice (remaining as they are or making some change). It can also be helpful to break down the big choice into smaller ones. For example, it is possible to be 'out' in some places but not others, to make some physical changes but not others, or to start down a certain path (towards a name change or surgery for example) and keep tuning in to how it feels every step of the way, rather than assuming that embarking on that path means having to continue to the end of it. Buddhist mindful therapies can be helpfully woven together with existential approaches here, given that they share much in terms of philosophy, and they offer explicit practices to help clients to be present with themselves and to tune into their experiences compassionately (see Barker, 2013).

Similar to existential therapy, systemic approaches to therapy are very much engaged with social constructionism, postmodernism, and post-structuralism: all theories which question the idea of object truths and rather see all human experience as culturally and historically situated (e.g. a same-sex-attracted person would experience themselves in very different ways in times and places where this was seen as a sin, a crime, a sickness, or a personal identity—see Stewart, this volume). Therefore, there is real potential for systemic approaches to see gender as non-binary but rather a culturally, historically, geographically, and linguistically contextualised invitation, rather than as a natural and universal construct (see Vincent and Manzano-Santaella, this volume). The challenging—or deconstructing—of dominant understanding of masculinity and femininity may be useful for clients. However, it may need combining with more phenomenological therapy to encompass clients' own lived experience.

Systemic practitioners, such as family therapists, have the potential of applying these lenses in their work with individual clients and larger family systems across the lifespan (Iantaffi, 2014). For example, a systemic approach could support a therapist in viewing gender identities as an ongoing, negotiated invitation rather than a unified self-identification (Harré, 1997). The therapist could then invite the client to be curious about those moments when they are invited into a binary view of gender, and to explore how they might be able to respond to those invitations from a non-binary position. Systemic approaches, combined with a narrative approach (which focuses on how experiences unfold—and are told as stories—over time), can also be useful when working with families of young non-binary-identified people. The therapist can externalise both gender and cisgenderism as constructs outside the client, rather than purely internal, intrapsychic experiences. For example, an individual or family might even be encouraged to speak to the dominant binary understanding of gender as if it is a person in the room occupying an empty chair, or they could compose a letter to transphobia. Such approaches allow a family to consider their own relationship to those constructs and how they might be reinforced or challenged, their impact on the non-binary person, and to recognise the power of dominant binary discourses on the whole system.

To summarise the key practical points from this section; when working with non-binary clients we would advise professionals to:

- provide clients with a space in the therapy room which is open to—and affirming of—all gender identities and expressions.
- make an effort to educate yourself on these matters generally, and on theories and research in your particular therapeutic approach which are inclusive of non-binary experience (drawing on some of the resources mentioned here).
- be willing to sit with a client's uncertainty and anxiety about either making changes, or remaining where they are. Demonstrating to them that it is possible to stay with such difficult feelings can be immensely valuable, and it is vital that they don't feel rushed into any decisions.
- normalise clients' experiences and identities with reference to the research and/or media depictions of non-binary people. Encourage them to see any distress they experience as systemic and structural rather than purely individual: reflecting on how binary assumptions are embedded within their families, communities, and wider society.

Non-binary People and the Practice of Psychotherapy

To date, there is little specific evidence regarding the experiences of non-binary clients in psychotherapy. However, Harrison, Grant, & Herman (2012) found that 43% of their non-binary participants had been refused medical care more broadly. Also, anecdotally we have heard of many non-binary therapy clients who have sought out an explicitly trans-affirmative practitioner having encountered stigmatising and pathologising practices elsewhere. This is sadly unsurprising given the research on therapy with bisexual and trans clients which has found that many practitioners and services remain ill-equipped to work with clients who challenge binary understandings of sexuality and/or gender. At best, therapists expect clients to educate them and use terminologies which reflect implicit bias (see Moon, 2008; Richards & Barker, 2013); and at worst, they pathologise their clients' sexuality or gender, and/or endeavour to change it to fit a binary or cisgenderist model (see Page, 2007; Somerville, 2015). Non-binary identities are still not broadly seen as legitimate; and even social constructionist-oriented writers have struggled to dismantle a cisgenderist, binary construct of gender (Iantaffi, 2015).

Related to this, we would underline the fact that—as with all marginalised sexualities and genders—any non-binary experience will be unrelated to presenting issues for the majority of clients (Richards & Barker, 2013). Practitioners should not link the client's gender to their experience of, for example, bereavement, work-related stress, relationship problems, or other struggles, any more than they would with a binary gender client.

With most openly non-binary clients, the main task for the therapist is therefore to have a generally good-enough understanding about non-binary genders (of the kind that will hopefully be provided by this volume) in addition to the capacity to hold the same kind of awareness of the potential relevance of gender as they would for any client. That is to say that we *all* experience the world in gendered ways that impact our experiences, mental health, and emotional expression. Gender is part of the picture, as are class, race, ethnicity, cultural background, family norms, generation, age, dis/ability, and the like. If practitioners do *not* feel able to hold non-binary gender experiences lightly in this way, then it would be appropriate for them to refer non-binary clients on to a more affirmative practitioner until they have undergone more training and self-reflection on their own gender (Bornstein, 1998; Iantaffi & Barker, 2017, being great starting points for the latter).

This said, given the current burgeoning popular awareness of non-binary gender identities and expressions, it is likely that practitioners—particularly those with specialities in working with LGBT clients or with gender and sexually diverse populations—will be approached by non-binary clients explicitly wanting to talk about their gender experiences and/or identities. Given the limited amount of research in this area, it is useful for such practitioners to stay up to date with the current literature, particularly qualitative research on the lived experience of non-binary people (Richards, this volume). This will act as a useful reminder both of the common issues that non-binary people experience and of the diversity of non-binary experiences, particularly when we are mindful of the ways in which gender intersects with other aspects of identity and experience such as race, ethnicity, sexuality, age, class, dis/ability, and geographical location (see Vincent & Manzano, this volume).

Common Issues for Non-binary Clients

Here is a brief—and no-doubt incomplete—account of common reasons—in our experience—that non-binary people may specifically seek help and support from a counsellor or psychotherapist:

First, many clients want to explore possible changes they might make to the way they identify, and the potential implications of these. For example, clients may wish to consider the terminology they use to refer to their gender (NB, genderqueer, androgynous, gender neutral, bigender, etc.), their title (Mx being one gender-neutral option), their name (moving to a different, or neutral, name), their pronouns (moving to gender-neutral options such as alternating *she* and *he*, *they*, *ze*, or *per*), and/or the terms they want others to use in relation to them (e.g. *sibling, partner, offspring, friend*, and *folks*, being neutral options—complete lists of non-binary terminology and pronouns can readily be found online). They may wish to formalise these changes in paperwork as much as possible, so it is useful to know the current legal options in your particular location.

Second, clients may well want to consider possible changes that they might make to their appearance and gender expression. This might include temporary changes to clothing, accessories, hair and the like, and more permanent changes including body modification through surgical interventions, tattoos, and hormones (see Richards et al., 2015, for a detailed overview). There are also changes such as those to voice, posture, gait, and engaging in body modification through physical activity which fall between these poles of temporary and permanent. It is important to be mindful here of the differences faced by people assigned male or female at birth in terms of expressing non-binary genders. For male-assigned people, the smallest change such as wearing nail polish or jewellery may clearly signify gender 'difference'; whereas for female-assigned people, even wearing entirely 'masculine' clothes and hairstyle may not be enough to stop them being read simply as 'woman'. Of course both of these positions can be challenging for clients, in different ways. It is also important to be mindful of the impact of those changes on clients within wider trans misogynistic contexts; wherein femininity can still be regarded as somehow inferior to masculinity. Also important here is the fact that each client is likely to have a unique journey through potential changes with all different combinations being possible. It is useful for the practitioner to have some knowledge of what gender specialist services are available in their local area and further afield, and how a client could go about accessing these in order to work within a realistic sense of what the current possibilities are.

Thirdly, a commonly discussed issue is whether clients want to 'come out', or 'stay in' about their gender in specific, or multiple, places. Research has found that trans people in general adopt multiple strategies when it comes to how open they are about their gender and/or transition (Morgan, 2015). Again it is important that practitioners are open to all these possibilities rather than harbouring assumptions that it is 'better' to always be out, or necessary to 'pass' for example. The potential rewards and punishments of outness and in-ness will differ radically from client to client and across locations and intersection of identities (e.g. in LGBT communities; with friends; in the workplace; with birth family; for BME clients; clients with disabilities; etc.). Some will conceal their non-binary gender from everybody. Others will exclude themselves from situations where they fear it will not be respected. Others will negotiate outness across situations. Others will be open publicly, or across all situations in their lives.

Some clients will already have been through a binary transition (to being a trans man or woman given that—for a long time—this was the only available trans narrative) and will be negotiating a shift from that to a non-binary identity. This will likely raise different issues than those for whom the non-binary shift is their first transition. There will be some familiarity with the processes, but also perhaps some concern about how others will perceive a further shift. Others may have occupied a lesbian or gay identity—for example, as a butch woman or drag king, camp man or drag queen. Moving to an explicitly non-binary identity from such an identity can pose challenges such as some loss of the previous identity and/or loss of community support if such communities are transphobic or lack awareness of non-binary issues. Additionally, for some clients, a non-binary identity may be a stepping stone on the way to a transition to a binary trans status. It is important that we hold equally the fact that non-binary gender experiences, identities, and expressions can be both a journey and a destination.

Many clients may wish to talk about how they deal with specific experiences of discrimination and/or invisibility. For example, a client may seek support to deal with the fact that family, friends, or partners refuse to respect their identity and use appropriate terminology, including pronouns. They may want help with how to handle a lack of available support or services in their workplace. Or they could be struggling with explicit discrimination or bullying from a boss, neighbours, or strangers on the street. Generally speaking, practitioners can work with such issues in the way they would with any client, but ideally with a backdrop of knowledge on non-binary issues and explicit affirmation of the client's gender given the lack of affirmation that they are experiencing elsewhere. In some cases, practitioners can work directly with these matters in relationship or family therapy, for example. Systemic approaches, as suggested earlier in this chapter, can be particularly useful in those cases in order to invite the family to look at their relationships with the idea of gender, and to further explore how context, history, and experiences have impacted their understanding of gender. Such explorations can support the de-pathologisation of the non-binary client who might have been positioned as 'difficult, challenging and other' within their family system.

Through all of these issues, it is important to balance an acknowledgement that the problem generally lies with the binary gender assumptions inherent in wider culture; with a pragmatic recognition that the client—like all of us—does need to operate within this world; and acknowledging the longer-term potential for systemic and structural change. It may well be helpful to explore with the client the inter-relationship between the gendered messages that they receive from wider society, through the institutions and communities that they engage with, within their interpersonal relationships, and in their own internal thoughts (see Barker, 2015b). This can lead to a useful consideration about how they might hold their non-binary experience firmly enough to feel authentic, and lightly enough that they are not engaging in constant self-monitoring and self-criticism (e.g. in relation to internalised binary assumptions or cultural ideals about what a non-binary person should look and sound like).

To summarise the key practical points from this section; when working with non-binary clients we would advise professionals to:

* always adopt clients' terminology, asking them which they prefer, and simply apologising and moving on if you get it wrong. Be open to supporting clients to explore possible identity terms, pronouns, and other gender-appropriate language.
* be aware of options for temporary and permanent physical changes (and everything in between) and be open to discussing the implications of these with clients: what they might open up, and close down, in relation to their experience.
* similarly, be aware of the potential costs and benefits of outness; and be open to helping clients to explore these in relation to their own lives, mindful of their intersecting identities, their social context, and where they are coming from (in relation to previous gender/sexual identities and cis/trans status).
* be mindful of the wider cultural context in relation to gender in general, and non-binary gender in particular, and how this will impact on your client as they navigate visibility/invisibility, discrimination, and harassment.

The Process of Working with Non-binary Clients

Three further matters worth considering here are whether practitioners are open with clients about their own gender identities, how services are monitored, and whether therapy is always the most appropriate form of support.

Of course all therapeutic approaches have their own stances on therapist self-disclosure; however, it is worth being mindful that binary gender is often something that can be read directly off a practitioner by a client. For this reason, it may be regarded as important that non-binary therapists' genders are equally readily available to clients. For example, the genders of all practitioners in the service could be listed, or they could employ an email signature which includes their pronouns. However, of course, not all practitioners will be comfortable with that level of public disclosure given the current status of non-binary gender. Thus, it remains for each therapist to determine how and when they disclose, and about what—in the best interests of their client, ideally with supportive supervision as necessary. It is also important that cis and binary therapists routinely engage with practices such as making their own identities and pronouns explicit, in order to normalise that gender is a construct we are all engaged with, rather than expect only trans and/or non-binary identified practitioners to consider the impact of self-disclosure.

Similarly, it is useful to determine in advance how clients at a service will be monitored. It is important to have some sense of how many non-binary clients are accessing services for equality and diversity reasons. However, again, people should not be forced into a position of disclosing their gender if they are uncomfortable doing so. Generally speaking, either an open box regarding gender or at least an *other* option in addition to *male/female* is appropriate, along with a *don't know/prefer not to say* option. An option to provide the name and pronouns that the client would like to be used seems essential for all clients to feel welcome and for practitioners to approach clients respectfully and competently.

Finally, it is useful for practitioners to be aware of available alternatives to conventional therapy such as community support and engagement with online resources. Sometimes, supportive groups with diverse and related experiences can be more helpful than one-to-one therapy (Barker, 2010), and many clients find it useful to engage with online materials and online and offline groups about non-binary gender in order to find support and ways of making sense of their experience. For example, in the UK, the Beyond the Binary website includes information, role models, and a non-binary agony uncle (see Bergman, this volume, for further examples). However, many clients may feel they want to find their own way and/or have little interest in engaging with non-binary communities, particularly if they view their gender more as experience than identity, or have a reluctance to foreground this aspect of their experience. Other aspects of a client's identities might also impact those choices, for example their dis/ability status, race and ethnicity, as well as class, age, and sex assigned at birth. All these identities will impact upon access to, and interactions with, non-binary communities.

To summarise the key practical points from this section, we would advise, when working with non-binary clients, to:

- undertake reflexive work around your own gender identity, experience, and assumptions, and consider where you stand on the ethics of self-disclosure in therapy.
- ensure that all client monitoring in your service is fully inclusive of non-binary people, as well as any materials that are available to clients, toilets on site, visual imagery online and offline, etc.
- be aware of any local, national, and international non-binary and genderqueer communities (online and offline) which might be useful points of support for clients, as well as being open to the fact that these may be more inclusive of some clients than others.
- in addition, encourage other staff in your services to make themselves aware, or undertake training, in these areas. Be prepared to explain the situation when communicating with other services if people are misgendering clients or otherwise demonstrating lack of understanding.

Summary

To summarise this chapter, non-binary affirmative therapy involves the following elements (see Richards & Barker, 2013, for further details):

- Being open to the diversity of non-binary identities and experiences, to the centrality—or not—of gender in each person's life and how it intersects with other elements and identities, and to the range of options non-binary people may want to consider in relation to their own gender.
- Understanding the potential links between non-binary gender and mental health issues via wider cultural invisibility and stigmatisation, as well as recognising the potential mental health benefits of non-binary experience and the lack of any necessary connection between non-binary genders and presenting therapeutic issues.
- Having reflexively explored one's own gender identities and experiences, and critically engaged with any binary—and other gender—assumptions inherent in your therapeutic approach.
- Being aware of key issues facing non-binary people including identity, physical changes and other aspects of transition, coming out/staying in, and dealing with discrimination, erasure and invisibility.
- Cultivating knowledge and skills on working ethically with non-binary clients, including correct use of names and pronouns, sitting with any uncertainty around potential choices, and affirming the client's lived experience of their gender.
- Educating yourself on referral routes in relation to gender services in your area, and being prepared to refer on yourself if appropriate (see Richards; Bouman, this volume, for further details).

References

Barker, M. (2010). Sociocultural Issues. In M. Barker, A. Vossler, & D. Langdridge (Eds.), *Understanding Counselling and Psychotherapy* (pp. 211–233). London: Sage.

Barker, M. (2011). De Beauvoir, Bridget Jones' Pants and Vaginismus. *Existential Analysis, 22*(2), 203–216.

Barker, M. (2013). *Mindful Counselling & Psychotherapy: Practising Mindfully Across Approaches and Issues.* London: Sage.

Barker, M. J. (2015a). Depression and/or Oppression? Bisexuality and Mental Health. *Journal of Bisexuality.* doi:10.1080/15299716.2014.995853.

Barker, M. J. (2015b). *Social Mindfulness*. Retrieved August 17, 2015, from http://rewritingtherules.wordpress.com/resources-2/social-mindfulness-zine

Barker, M. J., & Richards, C. (2015). Further Genders. In C. Richards & M. Barker (Eds.), *Handbook of the Psychology of Sexuality and Gender* (pp. 166–182). Basingstoke, UK: Palgrave Macmillan.

Barker, M., Richards, C., Jones, R., Bowes-Catton, H., & Plowman, T. (2012). *The Bisexuality Report: Bisexual Inclusion in LGBT Equality and Diversity*. Milton Keynes, UK: The Open University, Centre for Citizenship, Identity and Governance.

Barker, M., Vossler, A., & Langdridge, D. (Eds.). (2010). *Understanding Counselling and Psychotherapy*. London: Sage.

Barker, M.-J., & Scheele, J. (2016). *Queer: A Graphic History*. London: Icon Books.

Bem, S. L. (1995). Dismantling Gender Polarization and Compulsory Heterosexuality: Should We Turn the Volume Down or Up? *Journal of Sex Research, 32*(4), 329–334.

Bem, S. L., & Lenney, E. (1976). Sex Typing and the Avoidance of Cross-Sex Behavior. *Journal of Personality and Social Psychology, 33*(1), 48.

Bornstein, K. (1998). *My Gender Workbook*. London: Routledge.

Davies, D., & Barker, M. J. (2015). How GSD is Your Therapy Training? *The Psychotherapist, 16*(Autumn), 8–10.

Fine, C. (2010). *Delusions of Gender: How Our Minds, Society, and Neurosexism Create Difference*. New York: WW Norton & Company.

Harré, R. (1997). *The Singular Self: An Introduction to the Psychology of Personhood*. London: Sage.

Harrison, J., Grant, J., & Herman, J. L. (2012). *A Gender Not Listed Here: Genderqueers, Gender Rebels, and Otherwise in the National Transgender Discrimination Survey*. Los Angeles: eScholarship, University of California.

Iantaffi, A. (2014). Family Therapy and Sexuality: Liminal Possibilities Between Systemic and Existential Approaches. In M. J. Milton (Ed.), *On Sexuality: Existential Perspectives on Psychotherapy, Sexuality and Related Experiences*. Ross-on-Wye, UK: PCCS Books.

Iantaffi, A. (2015). Gender and Sexual Legitimacy. *Current Sexual Health Reports, 7*(2), 103–107.

Iantaffi, A., & Barker, M.-J. (2017). *Gender: A Guide for Every Body*. London: Jessica Kingsley.

Iantaffi, A., & Bockting, W. O. (2011). Views from Both Sides of the Bridge? Gender, Sexual Legitimacy and Transgender People's Experiences of Relationships. *Culture, Health & Sexuality, 13*(3), 355–370.

Lenihan, P., Kainth, T., & Dundas, R. (2015). Trans Sexualities. In C. Richards & M. Barker (Eds.), *Handbook of the Psychology of Sexuality and Gender* (pp. 129–147). Basingstoke, UK: Palgrave Macmillan.

McNeil, J., Bailey, L., Ellis, S., Morton, J., & Regan, M. (2012). *Trans Mental Health Study 2012*. Retrieved June 13, 2014, from http://www.scottishtrans.org

METRO Youth Chances. (2014). *Youth Chances Summary of First Findings: The Experiences of LGBTQ Young People in England*. London: METRO.

Moon, L. (Ed.). (2008). *Feeling Queer or Queer Feelings*. London: Routledge.

Morgan, E. (2015, May 29). *Trans People's Everyday Experiences of Managing Marginalised Identity*. Presentation to the Transology Research Event, London South Bank University.

Murjan, S., & Bouman, W. P. (2015). Transgender: Living in a Gender Different from that Assigned at Birth. In C. Richards & M. Barker (Eds.), *Handbook of the Psychology of Sexuality and Gender* (pp. 198–215). Basingstoke, UK: Palgrave Macmillan.

Nodin, N., Peel, E., Tyler, A. & Rivers, I. (2015). *The RaRE Research Report*. PACE. Retrieved October 21, 2015, from http://www.pacehealth.org.uk/files/1614/2978/0087/RARE_Research_Report_PACE_2015.pdf

Page, E. (2007). Bisexual Women's and Men's Experiences of Psychotherapy. In B. A. Firestein (Ed.), *Becoming Visible: Counseling Bisexuals Across the Lifespan* (pp. 52–71). New York: Columbia University Press.

Richards, C. (2011). Transsexualism and Existentialism. *Existential Analysis, 22*(2), 272–279.

Richards, C. (2017). *Trans and Sexuality—An Existentially-Informed Ethical Enquiry with Implications for Counselling Psychology*. London: Routledge.

Richards, C., & Barker, M. (2013). *Sexuality and Gender for Mental Health Professionals: A Practical Guide*. London: Sage.

Richards, C., Bouman, W. P., Seal, L., Barker, M. J., Nieder, T. O., & T'Sjoen, G. (2015). Non-Binary or Genderqueer Genders. *International Review of Psychiatry, 28*(1), 95–102.

Somerville, C. (2015). *Unhealthy Attitudes: The Treatment of LGBT People Within Health and Social Care Services*. London: Stonewall.

Titman, N. (2014). *How Many People in the United Kingdom are Nonbinary?* Retrieved August 10, 2015, from http://www.practicalandrogyny.com/2014/12/16/how-many-people-in-the-uk-are-nonbinary

Further Reading

Barker, M. J., & Richards, C. (2015). Further Genders. In C. Richards & M. Barker (Eds.), *Handbook of the Psychology of Sexuality and Gender* (pp. 166–182). Basingstoke, UK: Palgrave Macmillan.

Kermode, J. (2016). Images of Non-Binary people: How Poor or Absent Representations of Non-Binary People Contribute to Poor Understanding of Lived Experiences. In P. Karian (Ed.), *Critical & Experiential: Dimensions in Gender and Sexual Diversity.* Eastleigh, UK: Resonance Publications.

Richards, C. & Barker, M. (2013). Further Genders. In C. Richards & M. J. Barker (Eds.), *Sexuality and Gender for Mental Health Professionals: A Practical Guide* (pp. 71–82). London: Sage.

Beyond the Binary: A magazine for UK non-binary people. Retrieved from http://www.beyondthebinary.co.uk

7

Psychiatry

Sarah Murjan and Walter Pierre Bouman

Introduction

There has been an evolution in thinking about gender. Individuals in western society who have transgressed the traditional boundaries of gender and sexuality have been thought about, studied, categorised, and treated by psychiatrists. Just as 'homosexuality' was declassified as a mental disorder, so psychiatrists have come to see that transgender identities are not mental disorders, a view that is likely to lead to declassification of 'transsexualism' as a mental disorder in the forthcoming World Health Organization's (WHO) International Classification of Diseases (ICD) version 11, which will replace the current ICD 10 (Drescher, Cohen-Kettenis & Winter, 2012; WHO, 1992). As understanding with regard to transgender identities has increased, there has been an awareness of a proportion of individuals identifying outside of the gender binary.

S. Murjan (✉) • W.P. Bouman
Nottingham Center for Transgender Health, Nottingham,
Nottinghamshire, UK

© The Author(s) 2017
C. Richards et al. (eds.), *Genderqueer and Non-Binary Genders*, Critical and Applied
Approaches in Sexuality, Gender and Identity, DOI 10.1057/978-1-137-51053-2_7

125

There has been an argument that as the gender dichotomy has been challenged and non-binary experiences become apparent, gender should become largely irrelevant. However, the alternative view is that gender is diverse and consists of many more categories than the male/female dichotomy (Barker, & Richards, 2015). As there is no evidence that having a transgender or non-binary gender identity is a mental disorder in any way (Richards et al., 2016), it could be argued that gender diversity is not the business of psychiatry at all. It is also true that psychiatrists have attempted to treat gender-non-conforming people in a way that has not affirmed their identities and has been damaging, which has left a legacy of distrust for some communities. Specific psychological assistance for transgender people, including non-binary-identified people, may be delivered by psychologists, psychiatrists, and other mental health professionals. Expertise in the healthcare of trans and non-binary people crosses a wide variety of disciplines, and gender specialists may come from a variety of professional backgrounds. Psychiatrists still play a central role in the United Kingdom alongside psychologists and other health professionals in the assessment of those individuals who may be considering treatments such as hormones and surgeries in relation to their gender identity (Wylie et al., 2014).

There are important reasons why all psychiatrists should have an understanding of transgender and non-binary identities. Transgender and non-binary identifying individuals face particular pressures which may cause or exacerbate mental health difficulties. Prejudice and discrimination due to being a member of a marginalised group in society create marginalisation stress, which results in higher rates of anxiety, depression, deliberate self-harm, and suicidality (Haas et al., 2010). However, it is also really important to recognise that an individual's mental health difficulties may be independent of their gender identity as linking the two unnecessarily where it is not relevant to do so may be pathologising and stigmatising. All psychiatrists should have a basic level of awareness to enable them to communicate effectively with trans and non-binary people so as not to alienate and disadvantage their treatment. Access to services for non-binary-identified individuals is a real issue with many individuals being reluctant to come forward for healthcare or experiencing either discrimination or misunderstanding when they do so (McNeil, Bailey,

Ellis, Morton, & Regan, 2012; Whittle, Turner, & Al-Alami, 2007). It behoves all psychiatrists, therefore, to ensure that the services they offer are as inclusive and supportive as possible and for all staff to have a baseline level of awareness.

The Psychiatric Classification of Trans and Non-binary People

Gender diversity has existed across cultures and across time with numerous descriptions of gender-non-conforming people who have often had respected and specific roles within society (Nanda, 1998, 2008). There have been different ways of thinking about gender diversity which have been influenced by cultural and religious beliefs. Western monotheistic cultures have historically had an emphasis on sex for procreation and have viewed gender non-conformity and diversity of sexuality as sinful. Men and women were seen as separate and opposite. Scientific investigation in the late nineteenth and twentieth centuries challenged this view as Darwin came to prominence and embryology studies emphasised communal aspects of sexual development. Around the same time, Richard von Krafft-Ebing, a psychiatrist, published his study of human sexual behaviour in *Psychopathia Sexualis* (1886). He viewed homosexuality and bisexuality as perversions and described individuals who dressed as members of the opposite sex and believed themselves to be members of the opposite sex, viewing them as deluded.

Psychiatrists have continued to think about and classify gender and sexual diversity. As medical treatments, such as hormones and surgery, became available, trans people began pursuing physical treatments to align their bodies with their gender identity. Psychiatrists became involved in the assessment and care of transgender people seeking physical treatments such as hormones and surgery, and their role was enshrined in the Harry Benjamin International Gender Dysphoria Association (HBIGDA) Standards of Care documents (Benjamin, 1966). Diagnostic criteria were written for the diagnosis of 'Transsexualism' in the International Classification of Diseases (ICD-9; WHO, 1978) and 'Gender Identity Disorder' in the American Psychiatric Association (APA) Diagnostic and

Statistical Manual of Mental Disorders (DSM-III; APA, 1980). These criteria focused on identity of an opposite gender.

As more evidence has been gathered regarding the genetic, developmental, and hormonal influences in the aetiology of trans identities (Cohen-Kettenis & Gooren, 1999), psychiatric thinking has moved away from traditional theories, including neurosis in relation to oedipal concerns, castration complexes, and 'faulty' identification (Fenichel, 1930; Segal, 1965). There have been repeated calls from trans communities and from professionals for the declassification of trans identities as mental disorders (e.g. Global Action for Trans* Equality— GATE, and the International Campaign Stop Trans Pathologisation). Evidence that being trans is not a mental disorder (Richards et al., 2015), although may be associated with mental distress, led to the APA revising the diagnostic category in its fifth edition of the DSM (APA, 2013), replacing the diagnostic category *Gender Identity Disorder* with the category *Gender Dysphoria*, which emphasises distress as the core criterion. This was in response to calls for the de-medicalisation and declassification of trans identities, but also a concern that not having a diagnostic category at all might disadvantage trans people seeking medical care funded by insurance companies (Bouman, Bauer, Richards, & Coleman, 2010).

The WHO is also revising its classification of trans and non-binary identities. Their forthcoming 11th edition of the *International Classification of Diseases and Health-Related Conditions* (ICD 11), which is expected to be released in 2018, is scheduled to "declassify" gender dysphoria as a mental disorder; change the diagnostic terminology to Gender Incongruence; include non-binary people within this diagnosis so that those seeking medical care are eligible to receive treatment; and very likely place Gender Incongruence within sexual and reproductive health as a separate category (Drescher et al., 2012). This will lead to the rather incongruous and unsatisfactory situation that trans people, including non-binary people, fulfil diagnostic criteria for gender dysphoria in a psychiatric classification manual such as the DSM-5 in countries where they use the DSM-5, but also fulfil diagnostic criteria for Gender Incongruence, which will be classified as a medical condition (but not a mental disorder) in the ICD-11.

Interestingly, some Northern European countries, most notably the Netherlands, Belgium, and Sweden—which historically have been academic and clinical leaders in the field of trans healthcare and research—have moved gender identity services away from psychiatric services and into the departments of medicine (endocrinology). These developments will not only reduce stigma associated with being trans, but also serve as exemplary clinical service development models elsewhere (Arcelus & Bouman, 2016).

Psychiatric classifications and standards of care have emphasised the gender identity of the opposite gender with treatment to change the body to align with the opposite gender identity. The latest psychiatric classification, DSM V (APA, 2013), has worded the criteria in such a way as to include non-binary identities as follows:

4. A strong desire to be of the other gender (*or some alternative gender different from one's assigned gender*)

5. A strong desire to be treated as the other gender (*or some alternative gender different from one's assigned gender*)

6. A strong conviction that one has the typical feelings and reactions of the other gender (*or some alternative gender different from one's assigned gender.* (APA, 2013, p. 452f.; italics not in original)

As aforementioned, it is likely that the forthcoming revised ICD 11 will follow suit in this regard. Clinical guidelines such as those produced by the World Professional Association of Transgender Health (WPATH) have reflected the growing awareness of non-binary gender identities in their latest standards of care, version 7 (Coleman et al., 2012).

There has been a clear shift in understanding of trans and non-binary identities with growing awareness of a spectrum of gender identities and expressions. Whilst trans identities and narratives have evolved and psychiatric diagnoses have lagged, the number of people identifying as non-binary has been growing. However, it has been difficult to gain an accurate impression of the prevalence of binary-identified trans people from those attending gender identity clinic services as traditionally treatment has been offered to those who identify as the 'opposite' gender. Non-binary-identified individuals may have not been offered a diagnosis and treatment or they may have felt the need to fit themselves into the available [binary] psychiatric discourse in order to gain treatment. Clinicians will need to find ways to engage with transgender people to allow the expression of the full range of non-binary identities (Wiseman & Davidson, 2011).

The Prevalence of Non-binary Identities

As non-binary identities have become more recognised and treatments are adapted, it is likely that more non-binary-identified people will attend gender identity services requesting assistance and treatment. Although numbers of non-binary-identified people attending gender identity clinic services are relatively low, online surveys such as that done by Kuper, Nussbaum, and Mustanski (2012) give the proportion of trans people identifying as non-binary as approximately 50%. Again, studying an online transgender community, Iantaffi and Bockting (2011) found that approximately one third of trans-identified people did not identify as either male or female.

Population-based studies have estimated the prevalence of non-binary identities by looking at those who report an ambivalent gender identity, which is defined as equal identification with other sex as with sex assigned at birth, and those reporting an incongruent gender identity, which is defined as stronger identification with other sex than with sex assigned at birth. Kuyper and Wijsen (2014) found that 4.6% of birth-assigned males and 3.2% of birth-assigned females reported an ambivalent gender identity and 1.1% of birth-assigned males and 0.8% of birth-assigned females reported an incongruent gender identity, whilst Van Caenegem et al. (2015) found gender ambivalence in 2.2% of birth-assigned males and 1.9% of birth-assigned females whilst gender incongruence was found in 0.7% of birth-assigned males and 0.6% of birth-assigned females. This does not mean that these individuals experienced distress or sought treatment. Kuyper and Wijsen (2014) combined those with an ambivalent gender identity and those with an incongruent gender identity who also experienced a dislike of their gendered body and had a wish for either hormones and surgery, or hormones and surgery. He found 0.6% of birth-assigned males and 0.2% of birth-assigned females came into this category.

As the numbers of non-binary people in population studies are considerably higher than prevalence rates estimated from attendance at gender clinics or other health services (Arcelus et al., 2015), it is likely that the true prevalence of gender dysphoria is much higher than has so far been estimated and that the numbers of people presenting with non-binary identities are likely to rise considerably as services adapt their treatment to suit individuals with non-binary identities (Richards et al., 2016).

Relationship Between Non-binary Gender Identities and Trans Binary Identities

It is important to recognise that some people who identify as non-binary also identify as trans, but some do not. Some non-binary individuals may present to professionals as trans men and women because they believe that they are more likely to receive treatment such as hormones and surgeries.

In the past, when trans people underwent treatment in gender identity clinics, they went through a standard treatment that involved hormones followed by surgery. There was a heteronormative assumption that people fall into distinct and separate genders with different roles in life, with an assumption of heterosexuality as the 'norm' (Ekins, 2005). Trans people were required to complete such treatments or else face a lack of legal protection and recognition. Over time, there have been many more trans people having some treatments such as hormones without wanting other treatments such as surgeries or vice versa. Some have not wanted physical treatments at all, but want to be recognised as their experienced gender. These have sometimes been referred to as 'partial' treatment requests. A small proportion of these individuals have reported a non-binary gender identity (Beek et al., 2015), although it should not be assumed that, because an individual does not wish to undergo both hormone and surgical treatment, they have a non-binary gender identity. There may be many reasons for 'partial' treatment requests, including physical health issues, concerns regarding fertility, or concerns regarding surgical outcomes. Some people may feel that their dysphoria is relieved well enough following 'partial' treatment.

Whilst many trans-identified individuals may have had feelings about their gender and body from childhood or for some time, there is a process of gender identity formation that the individual undergoes. They may feel distress in relation to their body and feel that their experience does not match their peers in terms of relationships, gendered roles, and expression. This may lead to questioning and exploration followed by the discovery of a trans label and identification with trans people.

Non-binary-identified people may similarly experience incongruence between their gender, body, and birth-assigned sex. They may identify as either non-binary or trans and may experience their gender as fixed or fluid. For some binary trans people, there may be an initial identification with a non-binary identity. Others may go from a binary trans identity to a non-binary identity. This could be metaphorically likened to people who identify as straight, lesbian, or gay developing a bisexual identity or those who identify as bisexual developing a straight, lesbian, or gay identity.

There may be a particular difficulty for non-binary-identified people growing up, in that they may feel unable to identify with cisgender, trans male, or trans female role models, and lack of non-binary visibility may leave them without role models they can identify with. In these circumstances, non-binary individuals may be more likely to identify as either cisgender or trans and to try to fit into available roles. When they do discover the non-binary label, they may experience rejection and hostility from both cisgender and trans quarters.

Relationship Between Non-binary Identities and Mental Illness and Neuroatypicality

As with trans identities, there is no evidence to suggest that those with non-binary identities are any more likely to suffer or be diagnosed with major mental illnesses such as schizophrenia, major affective disorders, or personality disorders, although transgender people are over-represented amongst people on the autistic spectrum (De Vries, Noens, Cohen-Kettenis, Van Berckelaer-Onnes, & Doreleijers, 2010; Glidden, Bouman, Jones, & Arcelus, 2016) and this includes non-binary presentations. However, non-binary-identified people experience high levels of mental health difficulties and distress just as trans-identified people do (McNeil et al., 2012). This is complicated by evidence from McNeil et al. (2012) that trans and non-binary-identified people are likely to hide evidence of mental illness from gender specialist clinicians for fear that this will impact on their assessment for treatments such as hormones and surgery and are reluctant to come forward for psychiatric treatment for fear that they will be misunderstood or asked inappropriate questions; or that their gender will be focused on unduly. Given that 43% of non-binary-identified people have reported that they have attempted suicide at some point (Harrison, Grant, & Herman, 2012), this is concerning and suggests that they are not receiving appropriate treatment, which may lead to chronic mental health difficulties.

Suicidality amongst transgender individuals has been linked to younger age, parental rejection, and adverse employment circumstances (Haas et al., 2010). Similarly, the rate of non-suicidal self-injury is high amongst young transgender people (Claes et al., 2015). Mental distress has been linked to gender-based discrimination and victimisation (Clements-Nolle et al., 2006) which is often termed minority stress. Harrison (2012) found that non-binary people reported higher levels of physical and sexual assault than trans men and women. Baams, Beek, Hille, Zevenbergen, and Bos (2013) reported lower levels of psychological well-being amongst gender-non-conforming young people which were related to perceived experiences of stigmatisation. Non-binary people experience invisibility as there is little general awareness and understanding of non-binary people, and living in a non-binary social gender role in a binary gendered society creates issues which can be tiresome. There may be lack of understanding and inclusion from both cisgender and transgender quarters, and where there has been a shift from a trans to a non-binary identity, there may be rejection from trans-identified people who previously supported the person. Trans- and non-binary-identified people are more likely to experience lack of social support and to experience harassment and discrimination (Davey, Bouman, Arcelus, & Meyer,

2014; Factor & Rothblum, 2008). Additionally, non-binary-identified individuals may face greater barriers to access to gender services as well as difficulties in accessing healthcare in general in healthcare systems which are often inflexible and often provide gender-specific services and where professionals may have little or no awareness of non-binary identities.

Whilst non-binary identities may not be particularly *associated* with major mental illness, such individuals may suffer from major mental illness like anyone else. It is important for health professionals to be aware of the issues facing non-binary-identified individuals and to have knowledge of how to address and respectfully treat such individuals. However, as tempting as it may be, undue attention should not be given to the gender identity which may well be coincidental to the presenting mental illness. As well as perhaps being unwelcome for the individual, such undue attention may lead to the treating professionals being distracted from providing the most appropriate treatment and care (Richards et al., 2016). Nonetheless, some non-binary-identified individuals may present to mental health professionals with distress or anxiety around their gender identity. This is discussed further in the following section and in Barker and Iantaffi in this volume and Richards in this volume.

Psychiatric Evaluation of Non-binary Identities

There is evidence to suggest that waiting for assessment increases mental health issues, distress, and suicidality (McNeil, 2012); therefore, it is important that non-binary-identified individuals are able to access services promptly when they request them. To this end, further work to raise awareness of these issues amongst health professionals should be done so that patients can be referred appropriately without unnecessary delay. However, many gender services are struggling to deal with the rapidly rising numbers of referrals for treatment which may impact on waiting times.

Services should be explicit in welcoming non-binary identities as there may be assumptions around lack of availability of treatment for non-binary-identified individuals versus binary trans-identified individuals. Care should be taken not to pathologise non-binary identities and 'partial treatments'. However, it may be appropriate to question binary trans identities in some individuals who are not familiar with the concept of non-binary identities and may assume that they need to fit themselves into a binary identity.

It is important for professionals to be aware of the language associated with non-binary identities and to respect the individual's preferred pronouns and name. As there is no objective test, the diagnosis of a transgender identity, including a non-binary identity, is largely a self-diagnosis or identification. The history will often point to gender atypical behaviour from early childhood with growing dysphoria with regards to gender role and male or female secondary sexual characteristics. However, some do not recall a childhood history which is sometimes presenting later in life. What is more important than diagnosis is the assessment of the individual in relation to their gender identity, social gender role, expectations of treatment, and awareness of risks.

Whilst there is no evidence of a link between non-binary identities and major mental illness such as schizophrenia or major personality disorder, rarely such conditions will co-exist with a non-binary identity. It is also important to rule out extremely rare cases of people with such conditions who present as non-binary as a result of symptoms connected to their illness, for example, someone with schizophrenia who identifies as non-binary because of delusional beliefs that they have genitalia of both a man and a woman.

Levels of distress, depression and anxiety, as well as suicidal ideation should be assessed. Some individuals present with anxiety around their gender identity. They may wish to explore their gender identity or to consider coming out and making a social gender role transition. They will need to weigh up the potential gains and losses and to consider how they may wish to negotiate disclosure and transition in terms of their relationships with significant others and with wider society and work. A cognitive behavioural approach can be useful using a positive approach, mindful of the many non-binary-identified individuals who lead happy, successful lives. It may be appropriate for clinicians to meet with people in the individual's network to support them, listen to their worries, and facilitate negotiation between them and the non-binary person.

Some non-binary individuals will want to make a formal transition by changing their name, for example to a gender-neutral one, and by using a gender-neutral title and gender-neutral pronouns. This may present more difficulties in some environments than others; for example, using a title of doctor in academia may be less challenging than using a title of Mx in a shop. Further, more non-binary-identified people experience discomfort using gendered toilets than trans men and women (Factor & Rothblum, 2008). Evidence of a formal social gender role transition can provide evidence of a stable functioning gender identity. However, for a non-binary-identified individual, this may be quite tricky in societies that do not formally recognise non-binary identities.

Some non-binary individuals request treatments such as hormones and surgeries. These may relieve dysphoria in relation to their body and are treatments that give permanent changes that cannot be simply reversed. As many transgender people experience gender as fluid and evolving, it is important that the stability of the gender identity should be considered and where gender identity may be evolving or fluid, great care should be taken before recommending irreversible treatments. All individuals considering such interventions should be fully informed regarding the potentially irreversible effects which may be experienced. Generally, treatment for issues such as anxiety and depression should be given in parallel with treatments such as hormones as withholding hormones may exacerbate distress and damage the therapeutic relationship.

It is perhaps pertinent to consider that, as more evidence has emerged regarding the benefits of treatments such as hormones and surgeries for trans people with low rates of regret and adverse effects, the criteria for treatments such as hormones and surgery have become more relaxed and less stringent. Equally robust levels of evidence for those identifying as non-binary are not yet available and therefore there may be a greater level of scrutiny given to such treatments for non-binary individuals than for binary trans people. This may exacerbate the feelings of marginalisation that this group faces leading to poor engagement with services and potential for untreated health issues. It is important that services engage positively with non-binary-identified people giving them the available information to enable them to give informed consent to treatments whilst gathering evidence regarding the outcomes of such treatments.

Summary

Despite growing awareness of non-binary gender identities with growing numbers presenting to services with a non-binary identity, there is relatively little psychiatric research into the specific issues relating to non-binary identities. The paucity of specific research means that one must often turn to research regarding transgender people in general. This increasingly recognises the experiences of non-binary-identified people. Research needs to focus on issues pertinent to non-binary-identified people and their treatment without pathologising their identities. Psychiatrists need to become more aware of non-binary identities in both general psychiatric and specialist gender clinic settings. With growing numbers of non-binary-identified individuals presenting to services, psychiatric services need to ensure that they are affirming and supportive of them. There are difficult issues with gender-specific services, such as in-patient psychiatric wards, that will need to be thought about and addressed.

References

American Psychiatric Association. (1980). *Diagnostic and Statistical Manual of Mental Disorders* (3rd ed.). Washington, DC: APA.

American Psychiatric Association. (2013). *Diagnostic and Statistical Manual of Mental Disorders* (5th ed.). Washington, DC: APA.

Arcelus, J., Bouman, W. P., Witcomb, G. L., Van den Noortgate, W., Claes, L., & Fernandez-Aranda, F. (2015). Prevalence of Transsexualism: A Systematic Review and Meta-Analysis. *European Psychiatry, 30*(6), 807–815.

Arcelus, J., & Bouman, W. P. (2016). Current and Future Direction of Gender Dysphoria and Gender Incongruence Research. *Journal of Sexual Medicine, 12*(12), 2226–2228.

Baams, L., Beek, T., Hille, H., Zevenbergen, F. C., & Bos, H. M. W. (2013). Gender Nonconformity, Perceived Stigmatization, and Psychological Well-Being in Dutch Sexual Minority Youth and Young Adults: A Mediation Analysis. *Archives of Sexual Behavior, 42*(5), 765–773.

Barker, M. J., & Richards, C. (2015). Further Genders. In C. Richards & M. J. Barker (Eds.), *The Palgrave Handbook of the Psychology of Sexuality and Gender* (pp. 166–182). Hampshire, UK: Palgrave Macmillan.

Beek, T. F., Kreukels, B. P. C., Cohen-Kettenis, P. T., & Steensma, T. D. (2015). Partial Treatment Requests and Underlying Motives of Applicants for Gender Affirming Interventions. *Journal of Sexual Medicine, 12*(11), 2201–2205.

Benjamin, H. (1966). *The Transsexual Phenomenon*. New York: The Julian Press.

Bouman, W. P., Bauer, G. R., Richards, C., & Coleman, E. (2010). WPATH Consensus Statement on Considerations on the Role of Distress (Criterion D) in the DSM Diagnosis of Gender Identity Disorder. *International Journal of Transgenderism, 12*(2), 100–106.

Claes, L., Bouman, W. P., Witcomb, G. L., Thurston, M., Fernandez-Aranda, F., & Arcelus, J. (2015). Non-Suicidal Self-Injury in Trans People: Associations with Psychological Symptoms, Victimization, Interpersonal Functioning and Perceived Social Support. *Journal of Sexual Medicine, 12*(1), 168–179.

Clements-Nolle, K., Marx, R., & Katz, M. (2006). Attempted Suicide Among Transgender Persons: The Influence of Gender-Based Discrimination and Victimization. *Journal of Homosexuality, 51*(3), 53–69.

Cohen-Kettenis, P. T., & Gooren, L. J. G. (1999). Transsexualism: A Review of Etiology, Diagnosis and Treatment. *Journal of Psychosomatic Research, 46*(4), 315–333.

Coleman, E., Bockting, W., Botzer, M., Cohen-Kettenis, P., DeCuypere, G., Feldman, J., et al. (2012). Standards of Care for the Health of Transsexual, Transgender, and Gender-Nonconforming People, Version 7. *International Journal of Transgenderism, 13*(4), 165–232.

Davey, A., Bouman, W. P., Arcelus, J., & Meyer, C. (2014). Social Support and Psychological Wellbeing: A Comparison of Patients with Gender Dysphoria and Matched Controls. *Journal of Sexual Medicine, 11*(12), 2976–2985.

De Vries, A. L. C., Noens, I. L. J., Cohen-Kettenis, P. T., Van Berckelaer-Onnes, I. A., & Doreleijers, T. A. (2010). Autism Spectrum Disorders in Gender Dysphoric Children and Adolescents. *Journal of Autism and Developmental Disorders, 40*(8), 930–936.

Drescher, J., Cohen-Kettenis, P., & Winter, S. (2012). Minding the Body: Situating Gender Identity Diagnoses in ICD-11. *International Review of Psychiatry, 24*(6), 568–577.

Ekins, R. (2005). Science, Politics, and Clinical Intervention; Harry Benjamin, Transsexualism and the Problem of Heteronormativity. *Sexualities, 8*(3), 306–328.

Factor, R., & Rothblum, E. (2008). Exploring Gender Identity and Community Among Three Groups of Transgender Individuals in the United States: MTF's, FTM's, and Genderqueers. *Health Sociology Review, 17*(3), 235–253.

Fenichel, O. (1930). The Psychology of Transvestitism. *International Journal of Psycho-analysis, 11*, 211–227.

Glidden, D., Bouman, W. P., Jones, B. A., & Arcelus, J. (2016). Gender Dysphoria and Autism Spectrum Disorder: A Systematic Review of the Literature. *Sexual Medicine Reviews, 4*(1), 3–14.

Haas, A. P., Eliason, M., Mays, V. M., Mathy, R. M., Cochran, S. D., D'Augelli, A., et al. (2010). Suicide and Suicide Risk in Lesbian, Gay, Bisexual, and Transgender Populations: Review and Recommendations. *Journal of Homosexuality, 58*(1), 10–51.

Harrison, J., Grant, J., & Herman, J. L. (2012). *A Gender Not Listed Here:Genderqueers, Gender Rebels, Andotherwise in the National Transgender Discrimination Survey*. Los Angeles: eScholarship, University of California.

Iantaffi, A., & Bockting, W. O. (2011). Views from Both Sides of the Bridge? Gender, Sexual Legitimacy, and Transgender People's Experiences of Relationships. *Culture, Health & Sexuality, 13*(3), 355–370. doi:10.1080/13691058.2010.537770.

Kuper, L. E., Nussbaum, R., & Mustanski, B. (2012). Exploring the Diversity of Gender and Sexual Orientation Identities in an Online Sample of Transgender Individuals. *The Journal of Sex Research, 49*(2–3), 244–254.

Kuyper, L., & Wijsen, C. (2014). Gender Identities and Gender Dysphoria in the Netherlands. *Archives of Sexual Behavior, 43*(2), 377–385. doi:10.1007/s10508-013-0140-y.

McNeil, J., Bailey, L., Ellis, S., Morton, J., & Regan, M. (2012). *Trans Mental Health and Emotional Wellbeing Study*. Edinburgh, UK: Scottish Transgender Alliance.

Nanda S. (1998). *Neither Man Nor Woman. The Hijras of India* (2nd ed.). Belmont, CA: Wadsworth.

Nanda, S. (2008). Cross-cultural Issues. In D. L. Rowland & L. Incrocci (Eds.), *Handbook of Sexual and Gender Identity Disorders* (pp. 457–485). Hoboken, NJ: Wiley.

Richards, C., Arcelus, J., Barrett, J., Bouman, W. P., Lenihan, P., Lorimer, S., et al. (2015). Trans is Not a Disorder—But Should Still Receive Funding. *Sexual and Relationship Therapy, 30*(3), 309–313.

Richards, C., Bouman, W. P., Seal, L., Barker, M. J., Nieder, T. O., & T'Sjoen, G. (2016). Non-Binary or Genderqueer Genders. *International Review of Psychiatry, 28*(1), 95–102.

Segal, M. M. (1965). Transvestism as an Impulse and as a Defence. *International Journal of Psychoanalysis, 46*, 209–217.

Van Caenegem, E., Wierckx, K., Elaut, E., Buysse, A., Dewaele, A., Van Nieuwerburgh, F., et al. (2015). Prevalence of Gender Nonconformity in Flanders, Belgium. *Archives of Sexual Behavior, 44*(5), 1281–1287. doi:10.1007/s10508-014-0452-6.

Whittle, S., Turner, L., & Al-Alami, M. (2007). *Engendered Penalties: Transgender and Transsexual People's Experiences of Inequality and Discrimination.* Wetherby, UK: Communities and Local Government publications.

Wiseman, M., & Davidson, S. (2011). Problems with Binary Gender Discourse: Using Context to Promote Flexibility and Connection in Gender Identity. *Clinical Child Psychology and Psychiatry, 17*(4), 528–537.

World Health Organization. (1978). *International Classification of Diseases (ICD-9).* Geneva: WHO.

World Health Organization. (1992). *The ICD-10 Classification of Mental and Behavioural Disorders* (10th ed.). Geneva: WHO.

Wylie, K. R., Barrett, J., Besser, M., Bouman, W. P., Bridgeman, M., Clayton, A., et al. (2014). Good Practice Guidelines for the Assessment and Treatment of Adults with Gender Dysphoria. *Sexual and Relationship Therapy, 29,* 154–214.

8

Psychology

Christina Richards

Introduction

What is reality? How do we divide up the world into what is real and what is not? How do we measure what we find? In some sense, these questions have been key to psychology since its inception. We recognise the soul, the psy, at the heart of our science—but also strive for the rigour and the power which flow from the natural sciences; we try to weigh sadness on scales which would better measure out the nature of the planets, glaciers, or the flow of the oceans. Only at the sub-atomic scale do we have closer parity—a closer metaphor—with the human reality which concerns psychology; with things which may be both this and that, which may apprehend time in strange and unusual ways; which may bear ever closer scrutiny and yet still yield up insight into deeper complexity which is yet recognisable and representative of the greater whole.

C. Richards (✉)
Nottingham Center for Transgender Health, Nottingham,
Nottinghamshire, UK

C. Richards et al. (eds.), *Genderqueer and Non-Binary Genders*, Critical and Applied
Approaches in Sexuality, Gender and Identity, DOI 10.1057/978-1-137-51053-2_8

This paradox between the measurement of things with edges and those without sits at the heart of modern psychology and so inflects psychological understandings of non-binary and genderqueer people, as well as much else besides. How, for example, should we consider the ontology of non-binary people? As variation within either masculinity or femininity? On a spectrum between two 'poles' of male or female? As something entirely aside from the gender dichotomy? While our client's understandings are paramount and such considerations should be subsumed to them; the very work may consist of their seeking understanding alongside us. Indeed, the foundation of our approach, whatever it is, rests on an understanding of the nature of the presenting issue. For example, Cognitive Behavioral Therapy rests on a logical positivist assumption that *this* can be measured and that *that* intervention may change it by such a [Likert] degree. Phenomenological approaches, however—and especially existential ones—often frown upon fixed notions of identity; indeed fixed notions of anything aside from a very few existential givens such as Death; and yet many non-binary people do identify *as* such. Whether CBT, phenomenology, or any of the panoply of other modalities; it is the approach which invites the measurement, and so the understanding. Yet the measurement only captures a limited aspect of the phenomena in hand and so determines in that limited manner how it is apprehended.

Psychology then, as it relates to non-binary identities (as other identities), is in a bit of a pickle. So let's retreat from the swirl, ebb, and flow of the stranger tides of philosophy and onto the twin eminences of ethics and pragmatics—what are we actually talking about here?

Who non-binary people are has been eloquently discussed elsewhere in this volume, so we will not trouble ourselves to needlessly repeat that; suffice to say that there are many different sorts of folk—some who may identify as a static point on a notional gender spectrum; some who identify as a range upon that spectrum (gender fluid); some who have no gender (neutrois); and some who say Mu! (or *fuck you*) to the very question of gender (genderqueer or genderfuck people). The difficulty with the notion of a gender spectrum at all, of course, is that it assumes that the more masculine you are, the less feminine and vice versa. However, when you map traits or behaviours onto that, dyad things become more complex—if one is more aggressive, one is more masculine; less so, more feminine; but what of the mother defending her children? The father holding his new-born child? Aggression itself does not neatly correlate with gender, nor, indeed, does anything else. The gender binary and the gender spectrum become suspect.

And yet, and yet, we *do* have something called gender—we can perform the thought experiment in which we remove it from the world and see if the world remains the same: Remove jazz-loving penguins in fedoras from the world and it changes not a whit[1]; remove the internal combustion engine and it is unrecognisable—the former does not exist and the latter must do—even if we have no knowledge of what an internal combustion engine is or how it works. Therefore, we have *something* called gender; however, what it is, is complex and does not easily bottom out. But such is the case with something like music—for what makes music music? The Chinese peoples used to carry crickets in cages to sing to them as they walked—is that music to the [Western] modern ear, plugged in as it is to the electronic waveforms of recent music production? Those very waveforms too are a [binary] digital approximation of an analogue human vocal reality—the sweep and dip of the sine clipped to utilitarian ends.

But surely men and women are qualitatively, *quantitatively*, different—with different capacities and desires? This once seemed obvious, so obvious that women did not have the capacity to be educated; to vote; to undertake physical work; to be in the military; to be military auxiliaries; to be soldiers; to be front line soldiers; and so on. As we try to separate 'the sexes' to say nothing of 'the genders', we have to caveat more and more to retain the edifice we have built. We might consider giving birth to a child as a divider—but then there are trans men who have done so. Let us, as a thought experiment, exclude them for the moment: There are cisgender[2] women who have had a hysterectomy—are they female in this two-sex system? (Of course)—but let us exclude them too for now. Pre-pubescent girls—naturally they too are female, so let us exclude them as well in our ever-growing set of people who can give birth but who aren't female; or who can't but are. Those people who do not know if they can give birth? Those who opt not to? We must caveat and caveat to link being female solely with childbirth. What seemed simple is anything but. And we can do this with literally any trait: breasts? Mastectomy. Penis? Penectomy.

Consider chromosomes: We 'know' men are XY and women XX, yet ignore the fact that genes are expressed in complex ways—for the loss of function of RSPO and WNT4 genes causes sex reversal of an XX genotype to a male phenotype (without an SRY gene); indeed, overexpression of WNT4 or DAX1 also induces sex reversal. Additionally, changes in SRY and SOX 9 expression cause XY sex reversal (Whitehead & Miell, 2013). This is to say nothing of the role of post-partum environmental factors and epigenetic expression giving rise to a variety of body and neurological forms aside from a strict sex dichotomy (cf Joel et al., 2015; Joel & Fausto-Sterling, 2016). Even such things as strength which might seem self-evidently sex-linked are not always so; with right-hand average grip strength of people aged 30 to 34 not significantly differing between men and women[3] (Fain & Weatherford, 2017). Men do seem to do better athletically than women however; and yet take the best women rock climbers of today—send them back just 30 years and they will beat the best men—far too short a time to be an evolved difference. This is not to say that there is not a complex interplay of culture, genetics, neurology, and biology which give rise to some differences (as seen in the fact that women who inhibit expressed emotion score as well as men on that bastion of sex difference research, mental rotation tasks; Fladung & Kiefer, 2015)—but that these differences are far less robust than one might assume.

This complexity around strict binary sex differentiation troubles the traditional notions in psychology that men and women think differently as well as have different brains (cf Fine, 2011). There are, indeed, *no* psychological differences between women and men where the results are discreet. The overlap is vastly greater than any differences (when found, and as seen above that may be explained as an interaction in certain instances) and even then the effect size is minimal. Further, we know also that most psychological studies purporting to have generalisability to the [adult] population utilise a convenience sample of university undergraduates who are mostly between the ages of 18 and 22. While in most countries these people have reached majority and so are legally classified as adults, their neurological development has still not fully matured. Consequently, their brains are best characterised as 'late adolescent' rather than 'adult' as there is a deficit (compared to adults) in fronto-parietal activation implicated in control; and an increase (compared to adults) in ventrome-dial prefrontal cortex activation involved in emotional responses (Cohen et al., 2016). We also know that adolescents stereotype gender more than adults, both for themselves and for others (Alfieri, Ruble, & Higgins, 1996). Given there are observable brain differences between adolescents and adults, it is not unreasonable to assume that neurologically late ado-lescent college students may also have different responses compared to adults on [neural-implicated] tasks designed to discriminate between genders, especially those including stress, social behaviours, and inhibi-tion—that is, many of those given to undergraduates. That is to say that adolescent-brained college students may be demonstrating larger gen-der differences in tasks than an adult cohort would. Given the marginal power and effect sizes in many of the studies which purport to demon-strate gender 'differences', this calls into question the degree to which the adult population's performance on psychological tasks is actually split along gender lines.[4]

So, the emperor's clothes are looking rather thin, but we live in a world where most people do see them. Indeed, while we can reasonably confi-dently decouple gender from [biological] sex; and certainly challenge the notion of only a binary-sexed and a binary-gendered world; there does seem to be something called gender which is important to people and may have a neural substrate (Bao & Swaab, 2011). Note this is not about cognitive capacity differences, but about identity—which of course is inflected epistemically by social and psychological processes (cf. Richards 2017a). Consequently, there are people who have a certain birth-assigned sex and who feel their gender (for whatever that means to them) does not align with that sex; and further that their gender is neither male nor female. We might say that they are seeking certain bodily and psychic configurations which feel congruent. Some of these groups of people may be struggling to position their identity; some may have a firm idea of their identity but be subject to social pressures which cause distress; and some may wish to change their physical appearance though apparel and possibly also via hormones and surgeries. While the vast majority of these groups of people will not seek psychological assistance as they will be getting on with the quotidian realities of living; some will, and it is this group which we turn to now.

Clinical Considerations

As we have seen elsewhere, the evidence for the mental health of non-binary people is mixed, with some suggesting that non-binary people have raised levels of mental health difficulties (Harrison, Grant, & Herman, 2012) and some suggesting that the levels are the same as the binary trans population (which is still raised compared to the cisgender population—McNeil, Bailey, Ellis, Morton, & Regan, 2012; see also the introduction to this volume) and some suggesting it is less (Warren, Smalley, & Barefoot, 2016). Of course, mental distress in these groups is likely to be caused by minority or marginalisation stress—stress which is itself caused by social opprobrium and prejudice. Devoid of such opprobrium, it is likely that non-binary people would have the same rates of psychopathology as cisgender people—just as trans people do under those circumstances (Robles et al., 2016). Indeed, it is possible that non-binary people who are able to deal with external opprobrium may have the potential for better mental health than binary trans people as they must necessarily not have an identity which is compared against a [cisgender] norm—either by themselves or others.

Very often in my clinical practice I have a trans person, not uncommonly a trans man, who is determined that masculinising hormones will make them indistinguishable from a cisgender man. When I gently suggest to them that there may always be people who are aware of their trans status, they can be most discomforted by this. The difficulty is that they are trying to be something they can never be—a cisgender man. Note that I have not said they can never be a *man*—evidently they *are* a man, but they are a trans one rather than a cisgender one. Why should it be that cisgender is held as the standard of what a man, or a woman, is? As we have seen, these categories are broad enough to include [cisgender] older people; younger people; fertile people; infertile people; women with mastectomies and hysterectomies; men who have had penectomies due to cancer, and so on. Surely, they can encompass trans men and women too without breaking at the seams? Until trans men and women measure their gender by their identity, rather than an external cisgender [cultural] norm—which is often unattainable for many cisgender people too—there will always be the potential for mental health problems as trans people measure themselves and find themselves lacking. If non-binary people are able to ignore cisgender cultural norms as they necessarily identify outside of one side of the gender binary of male or female, there may be the option to avoid this stress altogether.

One may assume that it follows from this argument that it is therefore unnecessary for people to be trans or non-binary as the categories of male or female are wide enough to encompass a variety of gender identities and presentations. But I am not arguing that at all—quite the contrary. If we accept as axiomatic that there are two genders—male and female—(and as an aside this is, of course extremely open to debate) then it follows that there are people who feel they fit within them and those who don't. There are also those people who have bodily configurations they feel fit within them and those who feel they don't. There are those fortunate few—content cisgender people—whose bodies, identities, and cultural roles all accord and who do not need to do work to fit these together. However, these people are not the gold standard of gender configuration—they are simply a group of people who need to do less work to fit their gender configuration together.

Where non-binary people are especially at risk, however, is that their gender may be socially unintelligible (cf. Richards, 2017a) and so people find themselves in the trap of either seeming to be what they aren't and so being accepted, or seeming to be what they are and so facing opprobrium—a stressful situation felt by all minority groups with the option of concealing their identity down through the millennia. It follows therefore that any clinical approach used with non-binary people must not act like Procrustes, chopping and chopping until the client fits our, or our modality's, quaint notions of what people should be. We need to develop words and clinical frameworks beyond a gender binary or spectrum and beyond theoretical or modality stances if we are to respect non-binary people's identities and lives. In the meantime, ethics must trump philosophy (Richards, 2017a). Psychologists, scientist-practitioners as we are, can be overly theory-driven; while the theories we have are inadequate as they do not allow for an understanding of fluidity and fixity simultaneously and consecutively (cf Richards, 2017a). Be ware of the safety you find in your modality—while there may be dragons in the unknown; there have always been far more evil things lurking in the banal light of unthinking adherence (cf Richards, 2017b). What then are we to do clinically with our non-binary clients? Naturally, it depends on the understanding of the client and on their needs and capacities. Psychotherapy has been expertly covered here by Barker and Iantaffi, so I will not reiterate that here and I shall consequently focus on formal assessment of non-binary people, whether for referral for hormones[5] or surgeries; or for other purposes.

At the time of writing, determining the viability of a person for hormones and/or surgeries is often down to a mental health professional such as a psychologist. Historically, this gatekeeping role was fraught with difficulty, saturated as it was, in the trappings of modalities which did not recognise diversity in gender, or which pathologised it when they did. Consequently, assessments were lengthy and arduous as much attention was given to a person 'proving' their gender identity. Naturally from a psychological perspective, this sits uneasily as it disallows respect for the patient's autonomy and identity. We could argue (as many do) that any assessment of viability for physical interventions represents an undue imposition, but this extremely right-wing approach sits uneasily within nationalised healthcare—suggesting as it does that the Devil may take the hindmost—where the mistaken most vulnerable are seen as a sort of collateral damage to the easier path of the less vulnerable.

Having said that, there is of course an argument that this is just what we do with regards to pregnancy, where anyone may have a biologically related child—but there is far more screening for adoption. Further, we require crash helmets for motorcyclists, but smoking is legal. Our ethics relating to policy and law are not coherent and will doubtless be subject to change. Indeed, this relaxing of state imposition is often correlated with wider societal attitudes—just as with same-sex relationships, and then adoption and reproductive rights, things become easier as society progresses. That which was 'bizarre' becomes commonplace and no-doubt will continue to do so. One cannot help wonder what is next—perhaps trans-species where people identify as non-human animals? And recall that any negative gut reaction one may have will have been had in the past concerning other marginalised groups also. Ultimately, we need to respect autonomy and protect the vulnerable.

At least for now, given psychologists are required to make these decisions; how do we make them? The formal assessment given below gives basic information and a range of possible differentials. However, essentially an assessment of the viability of a certain person for hormones and/or surgeries consists of determining just two elements which, if you will forgive the idiomatic phrasing, can be summed up in just six words:

1. Is it non-binary?
2. Will it work?

This basically means determining (1) if there is some differential formulation or diagnosis which better accounts for the presenting factors, and (2) whether the proposed treatment is likely to be both benign and of some actual benefit to the client. Note that it's not about 'proving' gender—it's about matching the idea to the reality.

I hope that the future reader will forgive this focus on assessment—I believe such things as assessment (certainly as it is outlined here) will become an anachronism as the process of being comfortable in one's gender becomes a part of the ordinary flow of things. It would be nice if we could accept someone's gender much as we do their relationships—remarkable perhaps, but in the everyday sense of the word. If people want surgeries, then perhaps a greetings card?—as with a marriage or significant birthday—again notable, but as a part of the sort of things people *do*. Indeed, I'm sure my language will become archaic before a decade has passed. Please know then that the intent is noble—even if the sound to your future ears makes you wince occasionally.

Assessment then. A good basic assessment is below. Of course, first you will need a decent referral and will need to take account of any capacity and communication issues—certainly you'll need to tailor both the process and the content to the client and the degree of rapport. Remember some clients may well have had bad experiences with mental health professionals in the past and you may be starting in deficit as it were. Do also adapt it if you are not assessing for hormones and/or surgeries, although it can still be useful to find out about those things even if you are not—without focusing on them unnecessarily of course.

Ideally you should see the clients individually as they may be unwilling to answer questions about sexuality, money, and health with an intimate person present. If they ask for, or need the support of, another person present, then of course this must be respected. Under these circumstances, I sometimes say "I'm going to ask you about sex now. Are you still OK to have someone with you?", and if a good rapport has been established, they may ask their family member or friend to step out. Given the nature of the interview, I do not think it appropriate to have children present.

Assessment

Introduction

* What does the client want?

This can take some finding out, and a good answer is often "I don't know". Do get specifics—many clients assume everyone wants the same thing, when, of course, they don't.

* What is their gender identity?

Here, the heuristic of the gender spectrum can be useful (I often use birth-assigned gender as the 0 and the 'other' gender as 100)—is it a fixed point on a line from 0 to 100?; Is their gender a range on that line?; Something else? As stated above, the line itself is nonsense, but it gives a rough feel in the way a whale is 'big' and a mouse 'small'—even if they are not when compared to a planet or an atom. Having established what the person's gender is on this scale then, of course, you then need to find out what that actually *means*.

* What are their preferred pronouns?

Most people prefer *they*, but other options include xe/xyr/xem/xyrself, Sie/hir/hirs/hirself, and Per/per/pers/perself. Do respect this.

* Have they taken any steps to align their presentation with their gender identity?

This might include such things as identification documents with Mx instead of Ms, Miss, Mrs, or Mr; apparel; hormones; surgeries; and any change of name.

If people have made a change of name, it can be useful to find out why they chose that particular name.

If people are concerned about presentation, then graduated exposure can be useful. When people are catastrophising, it can be useful to bottom out the fear. "Everyone gets attacked and murdered" may change to "I always get attacked" to "I haven't been attacked, but my friend has, and I've been abused" to "I read about a person online being attacked and I think the people were shouting at me". This is not to say that non-binary people do not get abused—sadly it is all too often the case. But that there is a salience effect where people who are abused tell others; whereas people who have ordinary days don't—it's a bit like plane crashes; they happen, but only tragedies are reported and those tragedies unduly influence those who are prone to such influence—especially if that's all the exposure they have had to the phenomenon.

- Have they told anyone?

The most difficult people to tell can vary a great deal—some people's parents are very accepting, some less so; some children are fine, some less so. Work or education establishments can seem daunting, although increasingly have positive policies in place. Grandparents can be especially concerning as there may be ageist assumptions, but are often underestimated.

Younger non-binary people may not be taken seriously if they are not acting as adults in other areas—if their mum is still cooking, cleaning, washing up, and paying for everything while they play on their computer in their bedroom; then their mum may be more inclined to see it as a 'phase' than if the person is independent. In this case, the usual process of individuation as an adult may need to be managed alongside the process of coming out around gender; Some find a conversation to be a useful method to start the process of telling people, but this can be difficult between people with high expressed emotion; some find a letter where both parties have time to consider to be useful.

Of course, there are circumstances where one cannot tell certain people if there is a history of violence, for example. In these circumstances, families of choice and friendship networks will be vital. Do note that fear of violence can be as a result of tragic history and risk; or may be as a result of unfounded fear which can benefit from unpicking.

If they haven't told certain people there needs to be a plan—will they never see them again, ever? (What about religious ceremonies; birthdays; illnesses; funerals?) What would happen if their worst fears were realised? Their best hopes? That last is important too so as not to negatively bias the interview. It is extremely important for psychologists not to assume that living as a non-binary person is awful—it isn't. One can have a very happy life with a good career, children, partners, and so on (assuming one wants those things). It's not a matter of "well, you are this way, so you'll have to make the best of it"—there is much joy to be found.

Gender History

- How old when first disquiet or unease?

This gives a rough history, but people who have come to their gender later in life also go on to do quite well if they take things carefully and they rearrange their life gently and sensibly—without an undue assumption that surgeries and hormones will solve everything.

- How old were they when they first wore clothes not normally worn by that birth-assigned sex?
- When did they decide to change their body?
- When did they come out?
- Why come to me now?

Not uncommonly a life event has occurred such as leaving school; the death of a parent; retirement, a decade birthday, or the like.

Sexual History

- Have they ever had a sexual encounter?
- How old on the first occasion?

This can be useful to pick up any sexual abuse history—see below. It is also worth asking if they have had sexual encounters with people of different sexes—don't assume all partners will be binary or cisgender.

- Get a rough history of significant partners, including marriages/civil partnerships and the conception of any children.
- How does the person identify now in terms of sexuality?

I sometimes say—"How would you tick a box on a government form?"

- Are they using a body part they wish to alter currently?

If this is the case, then it is important that they consider the risks and benefits as well as just the benefits.

- Is there fetishism?

See *Differentials* below.

Family History

- Are they adopted?

This is needed to determine if there are any familial risk factors.

- Draw a genogram
- Physical and mental health of immediate family
- Any trans or non-binary family members?

As with friends, these people are usually (but not always) a helpful means of support.

- What was childhood like?

I usually ask this as "In a sentence or phrase describe your childhood"—otherwise, you may get the whole thing in a detail which is not wholly helpful.

* Any sexual or physical abuse?

I ask this separately and clearly, and very often get an answer that there was abuse even when told that the childhood was 'fine'. It should go without saying that there is no evidence that abuse 'causes' gender diversity; although it may inflect gender expression in some, extremely rare, cases. This should *not* be your first assumption (as you will likely be wrong).

Remember your duty to report if people are at risk. Remember you have a human in front of you who really, really needs you to be a decent human being at that moment.

Physical History

* Do they have any allergies?

If they want medical interventions, this is useful information.

* Do they take any medications?

It's worth asking about self-medication separately; as well as over-the-counter medications; and birth control as people don't tend to see these as 'medications'.

* Do they have any diagnoses?

I usually ask this as well as "Anything you see the doc for" as people with ongoing conditions sometimes miss things. I also ask it after medications as they remember those better than the diagnoses they are prescribed for. Pay attention to developmental conditions such as Autistic Spectrum Disorders (ASD); as well as strokes, clotting disorders, migraines, and psychiatric issues.

- Have they had any operations in the past?
- Do they have any Sexually Transmitted Infections (STIs)?

These may affect certain surgeries.

- Do they smoke?

This raises thromboembolic risk and can be a contraindication to some hormones and surgeries. People very often lie about how much they smoke. It's as well to explain the reasoning and to have some assistance available if they want to stop. Don't forget quitting is extremely hard and many people also enjoy smoking.

- Do they drink alcohol?

Aside from the physical factors, if people are having to drink a lot to mask their feelings, it can be difficult to get a read on how the transition is working out for them. The usual assistance should be offered if people are drinking to excess.

- Do they take illicit substances?

Similarly, if people are using recreational drugs, take whatever view you will. But if people need to mask their feelings that may need addressing, some people may have been using drugs to mask gender dysphoria—in this case, they should be assisted to move away from this coping mechanism when they are transitioning as the transition should act as a coping mechanism in itself (if carefully done) as the person comes to live in a way which is more personally congruent.

- How tall are they? How heavy?

A body mass index (BMI) over 30 can be a contraindication to some medical interventions. It can be extremely hard for people to lose weight—especially if they are using it as a means of masking a gendered body shape. I find it useful to encourage them to see it as part of a trajectory towards their goal—just as surgery is for some people—a painful interlude for a vastly longer benefit.

Mental Health History

* First contact with mental health services

Finding out if they have had contact with mental health services is useful—asking about counsellors specifically here can be helpful as people often think mental health means psychiatrists only.

* Get any diagnoses or medications not mentioned above.
* Self-harm and suicide attempts

Getting a rough history including deliberate self-harm and suicide attempts with predisposing factors and triggers is vital. Crucially, getting the date of last attempts is important as helping people is key. Also most important is assisting people to deal with triggers if they are stressed by, and during, a transition process. Remember, though, that you have a human in front of you—not a computer to be downloaded in the allotted hour.

* Get a mood score

I find a general mood score from 0% "The worst you've ever felt" to 100% "The best you've ever felt" to be useful to track progress. Note that this scale is relative to the person and not absolute.

Forensic History

* Get the index offence.

It is beyond the scope of this chapter to go into this in depth. Suffice to say sexual offences particularly complicate matters as the psychosexual process of the offender may affect their approach to gender. Of course, this is not invariably the case—offenders may be just as non-binary as anyone else.

* Get the sentence and (if in prison) tariff and likelihood of parole.

Again, this is complicated as there may be secondary gain in transition for people on long or indeterminate sentences. Some may feel that hormones or surgeries would appear to lessen their risk to the parole board (the risk is generally not lessened and may in fact be increased); Some may use it as a means of absolving themselves of blame: "I was only looking/touching the child to explore my own gender"—the criminal faulty problem-solving would still need to be addressed; and so on.

* Get key workers names.
* Assess risk.

The vast majority of non-binary people have never committed an offence. However, just as with any population—especially cisgender heterosexual males—some do perform criminal acts and should be treated accordingly.

Social Situation

* Find out where they live and if they are likely to be made homeless.
* Do they have any debt or savings?

You don't need to know how much—just if they have a means of support during transition or an additional stressor.

* Do they have supportive friends? Do the friends know about the person's gender?

For some non-binary people, as with some trans men and women, and especially when disowned or estranged from their blood relations—friends become a form of family sometimes called *framily*. This should be respected.

Educational and Occupational History

- Did they go to school?
- Were they bullied?

School bullying can greatly influence how people respond to the notion of transition, whether in school, just after, or far into adult life. If the person is in school, then they should be supported to get the school and carers to address the matter. Some schools are excellent at this; all should be. Just because it is in school does not make it acceptable—if you would not accept a work colleague doing it, then it is not acceptable in a school either.

If the person has left school, they should be assisted to recognise the differences in their adult life and to test out new responses to perceived threats.

- Did they graduate?
- What next? (University? Work?)
- Work history

This can be a useful marker of how chaotic people's lives are. They may need extra assistance with letters and appointments for example.

Formulation/Impression

This can include a diagnosis (BPS, 2012) such as gender dysphoria in the *Diagnostic and Statistical Manual* version 5 of the American Psychiatric Association (APA, 2013a) which specifically includes non-binary genders and recognises that they are not a mental disorder (APA, 2013b). However, this should only be used if absolutely necessary and for pragmatic ends. In terms of benefit to the client, my experience is that (aside from access to interventions) diagnosis does not assist.

Instead formulation is usually better employed (BPS, 2011), which succinctly identifies the client's current situation; desired direction and destination; and the strengths towards, as well as the blocks to, this occurring—whether psychological, practical, or both. Note, it's important not to confuse psychological and practical blocks—"Of course I can't tell my grandmother" might seem practical, but is likely psychological in nature. Similarly, "I'll be fired if I come out at work" may be entirely practical; but may be psychological—the more intelligent the client, the more intelligent their very sensible reason for not doing what they fear to do. Identifying the fear as well as the seemingly practical concerns can be very useful.

Plan

* Further sessions?
* Referral?
* Physical interventions?

Remember above all that this person is a human, a human who is suffering (thus they come to you—non-binary people doing all right won't be seeing you), and is a person who has likely suffered (or is certainly part of a group who have suffered) at the hands of mental health professionals. We need to be skilled, caring, and compassionate.

Considerations and Differentials

In the past, things were so wretched for trans people that only those who had literally no other option[6] came out—those people whose feelings were so strong and whose identity was so at odds with their birth-assigned sex had no choice. This group consequently opened themselves up to the travails being an out trans person entailed. This meant that many of those people were binary (they had travelled too far from their birth-assigned sex to hide it as 'tomboy' or 'effeminate') or if they were queer, they were so much so they too had no option but to be out. They were pioneers and we owe them an extraordinary debt for forging a path.

Things are still wretched in many parts of the world; but in some areas of the high-GDP West, there are spaces opening up for people to live outside of their birth-assigned gender which was not previously available. This means that people who may have previously felt they had to stay safe by nominally staying within their birth-assigned gender role are now able to come out. Thus, there is more of a mix of people with a range of degrees of gender dysphoria and a range of identities who are in the public, and clinical, eye. Similarly, there are differing amounts of bodily dysphoria becoming visible; and differing amounts of treatment seeking. These things are highly correlated—but not perfectly.[7] For example, you might have a person who is greatly distressed about their birth-assigned gender, but who does not desire physical interventions to change their body. Or a person with a mild dysphoria about their gender, but who especially dislikes their breasts. There are many non-binary people who have high dysphoria in all areas; but there are also people who have some aspect of dysphoria which is milder than that of the [mostly binary] people forced to come out who were referred to above. This is not to invalidate their identity—we none of us only do, and are, things we burn for—but it does make treatment decisions more difficult; and perhaps especially so when nationalised healthcare is involved in which psychologists must determine not only that the treatment is not harmful, but that it is of clear benefit.

In terms of determining likely benefit, differentials are, of course, vital in that physical or major social changes—if instigated for another reason than identity—may not turn out well. There are actually relatively few differentials one comes across in the general run of things. Far more often non-binary people are just that—non-binary—and should be assumed to be so. The differentials should be considered of course, but the non-binary person should only be considered not to be non-binary as a last resort. The main differentials are:

* Psychosis

This is easily addressed as those people who still have a gender identity which differs from their birth-assigned gender when their psychosis abates are like trans or non-binary and those who do not are likely not.

* Autistic special interest

There is a much higher rate of non-binary and trans identities among people on the autistic spectrum (ASD people; Glidden, Bouman, Jones, &

Arcelus, 2016), who will need the usual assistance afforded to neurotypical non-binary people but with appropriate accommodations being made. One key difficulty non-binary ASD people face is that they struggle with theory of mind. This means that they struggle to recognise that, while they understand they have a certain gender, if they do not communicate that fact to others—whether through apparel or other means—those others will not realise what the ASD person's gender is.

In addition to this group, there are a group of people, who are not trans or non-binary in the usual sense, but who have a special interest in gender and can become confused into thinking that they too are non-binary—especially if they have found a supportive (often online) group which encourages them in this belief.

* Fetishism

Many people feel more sexy in their [non-binary] gender of identity, rather than their birth-assigned gender, because they naturally feel more able to be sexual with an identity and/or body which reflects them appropriately. If there is fetishism or an interest in some aspects of BDSM as part of that, it may be that this is a safe place to explore gender.

Alternatively, there are those people for whom body alterations are a direct part of the fetishism (this is rare, but does happen). This can be a problem as once body alteration in permanent, the day-to-day familiarity removes the erotic charge leaving the person with no sexual motivation for the change; no identity motivation for the change; and an irreparably changed body.

* Forensic secondary gain

See *Forensic history* above.

* Immaturity

Some people who have yet to form a complete sense of themselves will try out identities to see if they fit. Thus, non-binary people may try out binary identities before settling on [a non-binary] one which fits.

Very often younger people will understandably look to their immediate social circle to try out identities. This is a natural part of adolescence and will include things such as sexuality and gender. There is no reason why a person should not try out such things if they include non-cisgender and non-heterosexual identities and practices as there is nothing wrong with a non-binary identity (or being same-sex attracted for that matter). It is not that there is nothing wrong (but being cisgender is preferred). There is simply nothing wrong. Period.

Having said that, it would be foolish to make permanent bodily changes which may be regretted under these circumstances, and so it is important to make sure the person is clear before making such changes. This is not to say children cannot be non-binary—they can—we just need to make sure that the identity is likely to be permanent before making permanent changes.

And:

* Non-binary identity as a path to a binary trans identity

This last is separated out as it is not really a differential by virtue of being something else entirely from non-binary; but more of a step on the way which is increasingly being seen as non-binary identities becomes more accepted. In this case, some people believe it is easier if they do not 'go the whole hog' and so they tell people that they are non-binary instead of transitioning into another [binary] gender entirely. Thus, if their name is John Doe, they may change to Jamie Doe and so avoid parental opprobrium as the parents can still think of them as Jamie (male) while their friends think of them as Jamie (non-binary). If they feel more binary gendered, this will not be entirely satisfactory for them and they then make a further change to a (in this case female) gender which feels more comfortable and so change again to Jane Doe and deal with any parental opprobrium. Unfortunately, and ironically, some people who opt for a non-binary identity as a means of avoiding opprobrium in fact find more—as at present many people expect a binary world even if some people have 'crossed the floor' between the genders. This can be the case even if the viewer thinks the person they are interacting with was assigned another gender at birth—it is still explicable within a binary worldview;

Whereas these viewers with a binary worldview can be more disquieted by people who appear to be neither male nor female.

Naturally, there are also some people for whom a binary trans identity is a step on a path to a non-binary identity also.

Psychologists may be especially well placed to undertake such assessments and consideration of differentials, given that they sit at the nexus of meaning, law, physicality, mental processes, and much else besides, and so may be more able to get to the heart of the individual in all their liminal, interstitial, psychically iridescent beauty. As we marshall this movement beyond the binary, however, we need to be mindful that clients may act as signifiers for a breakdown of social order linked to heteronormativity. When societies, institutions, and laws require a gender binary—in the form of single-sex prisons and changing rooms, for example—the political loading for societal change can rest on the shoulders of our clients, who may be especially vulnerable (cf Richards in Barker & Scheele, 2016). It behoves us therefore to advocate on our client's behalf, not only within the safe confines of our therapy rooms, but also in wider political arenas where our power may be brought to bear to affect societal change, rather than centring the need for such change within our clients and expecting them to carry the burden into the body politic.

We need to be especially aware here, as elsewhere, of the place of intersectionality. Where clients have multiple areas of discrimination or challenge, it is important not to silo each of these. What is true for a white middle-class heterosexual non-binary person may not be so for a working-class non-binary person of colour—there are very few matters which sit in isolation as 'non-binary matters' (or other matters for that matter—cf. Iantaffi & Barker, 2017). Consequently, advocacy might need to be in regard to social welfare, adequate housing, or the like, in order that the person can safely express their gender—to say it is not our business as "It's not psychology" or "It's not about gender" is to fundamentally misunderstand the interconnected nature of people's lives; and to abrogate the responsibility which comes with our roles as psychologists.

We need too to be aware of the role that gender is playing out in society—the meanings loaded upon it which it struggles to bear about power, possibilities, love, rights, sex, death—the stuff of life. We need to think about how people, including ourselves, may be policing one another's gender, and how we police our own as a sort of internalised panopticon with the inhered society always looking, pointing, criticising, and stopping who we might be were we to release ourselves. We need to strive to be all we can be; whether we identify within the binary or without, and to be kind and a source of strength for those around us who are similarly fighting that good fight.

Summary

* Reality is not binary—neither should our practice be.
* Be mindful of differentials while also supporting client's self-determination.
* Do use the person's preferred pronouns and name.
* The usual psychological assistance with anxiety; phobias; depression; relationships; bullying; and so on, can pay dividends with this client group too—even when the matter is apparently about gender.
* Be reflexively aware of what your own assumptions about gender are—whether you are trans, cisgender, non-binary/genderqueer, or anything else.

Notes

1. Sadly.
2. A cisgender person is a person who is content to remain the gender they were assigned at birth.
3. While other groups in the study did differ, this shows it is not *invariably* so.
4. I fear I shall have my psychology department tweed jacket's elbow patches ceremoniously stripped off for this heresy. Nonetheless, orthodoxies must be overturned if we are truly to be scientists.
5. As seen in in the endocrine chapters, a difficulty with hormone treatment at present, which may need addressing within the psychological consultation, is that, biologically sex development is 'opposite' for males and females to some degree; or Y shaped with divergent paths. There is complexity and variation, but one hormone or set of hormones often blocks

the expression of the other, thus a pure choice of body types is not currently endocrinologically possible. Consequently, attention must be paid to attributing comfortable meanings to extant body parts (body parts don't have inherent meanings) if they cannot be changed without a less desired change accompanying it.

6. Mostly, some of us were up for the fight to be ourselves too of course.
7. As a side note, this is the rebuttal to the incorrect assertion by some radical feminists and psychoanalysts that bodily changes would be unnecessary were trans and non-binary people to simply widen their understandings of gender. It is not that people are overly eliding physicality with gender—it is that people have a certain gender, and (independently and interrelatedly) wish to have a certain body.

References

Alfieri, T., Ruble, D. N., & Higgins, E. T. (1996). Gender Stereotypes During Adolescence: Developmental Changes and the Transition to Junior High School. *Developmental Psychology, 32*(6), 1129.

American Psychiatric Association (APA). (2013a). *Diagnostic and Statistical Manual of Mental Disorders 5*. Washington, DC: American Psychiatric Association.

American Psychiatric Association (APA). (2013b). *Gender Dysphoria Fact Sheet*. Retrieved November 27, 2016, from http://www.dsm5.org/Documents/ Gender%20Dysphoria%20Fact%20Sheet.pdf

Bao, A.-M., & Swaab, D. F. (2011). Sexual Differentiation of the Human Brain: Relation to Gender Identity, Sexual Orientation and Neuropsychiatric Disorders. *Frontiers in Neuroendocrinology, 32*, 214–226.

Barker, M. J., & Scheele, J. (2016). *Queer: A Graphic History*. London: Icon Books.

British Psychological Society. (2011). *Good Practice Guidelines on the Use of Psychological Formulation*. Leicester, UK: British Psychological Society.

British Psychological Society. (2012). *Diagnosis—Policy and Guidance*. Leicester, UK: British Psychological Society.

Cohen, A. O., Breiner, K., Steinberg, L., Bonnie, R. J., Scott, E. S., Taylor-Thompson, K., et al. (2016). When is an Adolescent an Adult? Assessing Cognitive Control in Emotional and Nonemotional Contexts. *Psychological Science, 27*(4), 549–562.

Fain, E., & Weatherford, C. (2017). Comparative Study of Millennials' (Age 20–34 years) Grip and Lateral Pinch with the Norms. *Journal of Hand Therapy, 29*(4), 483–488.

Fine, C. (2011). *Delusions of Gender: The Real Science Behind Sex Differences.* London: Icon Books.

Fladung, A. K., & Kiefer, M. (2015). Keep Calm! Gender Differences in Mental Rotation Performance are Modulated by Habitual Expressive Suppression. *Psychological Research, 80*(6), 985–996.

Glidden, D., Bouman, W. P., Jones, B. A., & Arcelus, J. (2016). Gender Dysphoria and Autism Spectrum Disorder: A Systematic Review of the Literature. *Sexual Medicine Reviews, 4*(1), 3–14.

Harrison, J., Grant, J., & Herman, J. L. (2012). *A Gender Not Listed Here: Genderqueers, Gender Rebels, and Otherwise in the National Transgender Discrimination Survey.* Los Angeles: eScholarship, University of California.

Iantaffi, A., & Barker, M.-J. (2017). *Gender: A Guide for Every Body.* London: Jessica Kingsley.

Joel, D., Berman, Z., Tavor, I., Wexler, N., Gaber, O., Stein, Y., et al. (2015). Sex Beyond the Genitalia: The Human Brain Mosaic. *Proceedings of the National Academy of Sciences, 112*(50), 15468–15473.

Joel, D., & Fausto-Sterling, A. (2016). Beyond Sex Differences: New Approaches for Thinking About Variation in Brain Structure and Function. *Philosophical Transactions of the Royal Society B, 371*(1688), 20150451.

McNeil, J., Bailey, L., Ellis, S., Morton, J., & Regan, M. (2012). *Trans Mental Health Survey 2012.* Edinburgh, UK: Scottish Transgender Alliance.

Richards, C. (2017a). *Trans and Sexuality—An Existentially-Informed Ethical Enquiry with Implications for Counselling Psychology* [Monograph]. London: Routledge.

Richards, C. (2017b). Starshine on the Critical Edge: Philosophy and Psychotherapy in Fantasy and Sci-fi. *Journal of Psychotherapy and Counselling Psychology Reflections, 2*(1), 17.

Robles, R., Fresán, A., Vega-Ramírez, H., Cruz-Islas, J., Rodríguez-Pérez, V., Domínguez-Martínez, T., et al. (2016). Removing Transgender Identity from the Classification of Mental Disorders: A Mexican Field Study for ICD-11. *The Lancet Psychiatry, 3*(9), 850–859.

Warren, J. C., Smalley, K. B., & Barefoot, K. N. (2016). Psychological Well-being Among Transgender and Genderqueer Individuals. *International Journal of Transgenderism, 17*(3–4), 114–123.

Whitehead, S., & Miell, J. (2013). *Clinical Endocrinology.* Banbury, UK: Scion.

Further Reading

Barker, M. J., & Richards, C. (2015). Further Genders. In C. Richards & M. J. Barker (Eds.), *The Palgrave Handbook of the Psychology of Sexuality and Gender* (pp.166–182). London: Palgrave Macmillan.

Barker, M. J., & Richards, C. (2016). Gender in Counselling Psychology. In D. Murphy (Ed.), *BPS Counselling Psychology*. Hoboken, NJ: Wiley-Blackwell.

Fine, C. (2011). *Delusions of Gender: The Real Science Behind Sex Differences*. London: Icon Books Ltd.

Richards, C., Bouman, W. P., Seal, L., Barker, M. J., Nieder, T., & T'Sjoen, G. (2016). Non-binary or Genderqueer Genders. *International Review of Psychiatry, 28*(1), 95–102.

Richards, C., & Barker, M. (2013). *Sexuality and Gender for Mental Health Professionals: A Practical Guide*. London: Sage.

Part III

Bodies

9

Child and Adolescent Endocrinology

Gary E. Butler

Introduction

This chapter discusses the biology of human sexual development at the different ages and stages, including male and female gender identity development, and diversity of sexual development and how this influences gender identity. It also discusses the effects of gender identity on the difference in the sequence of timing of the events of normal puberty in boys and girls and what happens when this occurs at the usual time. The effects of puberty and its blockade by gonadotropin-releasing hormone (GnRH) analogues and considerations of fertility preservation are discussed. Various hormonal therapies to attempt to reduce birth sex hormone production are rarely fully effective, and acceptance of this is variable.

G.E. Butler (✉)
University College London Hospital & UCL Great Ormond Street Institute of Child Health, London, UK

© The Author(s) 2017   **171**
C. Richards et al. (eds.), *Genderqueer and Non-Binary Genders*, Critical and Applied Approaches in Sexuality, Gender and Identity, DOI 10.1057/978-1-137-51053-2_9

Human Sexual Development

In humans, development of biological sex begins six weeks after conception. At that stage, under the usual developmental processes, there is a polarisation of sex development along a male or female line. Genetic triggers—in particular the SRY gene on the Y chromosome in the male assisted by a number of other autosomal genes—promote development of the primordial gonad into a testis containing embryonic sperm-producing cells, spermatogonia, and fetal Leydig cells which secrete testosterone over the ensuing 4 to 5 weeks. These genes, assisted by testosterone, transform the internal and external genitalia along male lines and cause disappearance of the female-associated structures such as the uterus and upper vagina.

It had formerly been thought that the default development pathway permitted the maintenance of the female urogenital tract, that is, vagina, uterus, fallopian tubes, and also the gonad remaining an ovary. We are aware now that there are active ovarian developmental genes as well, but there is no significant secretion of any hormone which alters the body systemically in a female pattern in the way testosterone masculinizes a male body.

The secretion of testosterone by the developing testis at 6 to 12 weeks of post-conceptual age masculinizes the internal and external genitalia and may contribute to male gender identification, although hormones are certainly not the only factor. When disorders of testosterone production occur, or where the action of testosterone is blocked due to partial hormone receptor defects; follow-up studies suggest that uncertainties of gender identity and non-binary gender identification are not the usual outcome despite there being physical ambiguities of the gonads and atypical development of the external genitalia.

Intersex/DSD and Non-binary Experience

What therefore is the outcome in terms of gender identity when there are congenital variations in androgen responsiveness which can also produce anatomical changes to the external genital structures? One of the more common forms of DSD (which stands for Disorder, or Diversity, or Difference of Sexual Development) is congenital adrenal hyperplasia (CAH). In CAH, biological females experience an excess of testosterone secretion produced by the foetal adrenal glands due to an autosomal recessively inherited block in steroid hormone production. Right from the start of organogenesis, the female embryo is bathed in high levels of testosterone, which can cause moderate-to-severe virilization of the external genitalia and, by supposition, the brain too. This potentially could cause a perceived gender ambiguity. There is even the rare situation where a female infant is assigned to the male sex on account of full masculinization of the phallus and labioscrotal folds giving the appearance of typical male external genitalia.

Much has been written about sexuality and gender identification of genetic females virilized from early on in life, yet male gender identification seems less common later on in life than would be predicted from the extent of the virilization. However, non-uniform female behaviour, that is, typical tomboy expressions, is frequently reported by parents of virilized female children with CAH in the prepubertal years.

The window of maximal androgenic hormonal effect seems to be relatively early on in life, that is, well before birth in the first trimester of pregnancy. There is also the well-recognised surge of testosterone reaching pubertal levels between 4 and 8 weeks after birth in male infants, sometimes referred to as a *mini-puberty* caused by a wave of the gonadotropins FSH and LH stimulating the testes to produce a level of testosterone of equivalent magnitude to that found at puberty. This blast of testosterone does not seem to have any known direct virilizing effect on male gender identity or sexual expression. It is absent in individuals who have abnormal pituitary development or lack pituitary gonadotropin secretion, and although spontaneous pubertal development and fertility do not occur in these boys, non-binary gender expression, or indeed any kind of gender dysphoria, is not the usual finding. So little evidence exists to suggest that a lack of testosterone has an altering effect on male gender identity development, whereas clinical follow-up studies clearly demonstrate that an excess of testosterone at key developmental stages may promote non-binary gender expression.

Environmental disruptors such as oestrogen-mimicking chemicals found in water as a result of industrial effluent and phenol-derivative plastic softeners commonly used in manufacturing such as polychlorinated biphenyls (PCBs) have all been linked to reduced masculinization. These include an increased prevalence of incomplete male sex organ development in fish and reptiles and possibly the rising incidence of hypospadias (incomplete closure of the urinary system in males resulting in the urinary opening being positioned below the tip of the penis). Environmental disruptors have been directly linked to falling sperm counts in humans over the last 50 years. Again, as with the hypomasculinization hypothesis, no link has been drawn as yet with non-binary gender expression. By contrast, however, as the use of certain classes of plasticizers in babies' bottles and children's toys has been withdrawn, non-binary gender identification has apparently increased, contrary to predictions.

Hormones and Gender Development During Growth and Puberty

There is little production of sex hormones in children after two months of age until the onset of puberty. The reproductive hormone axis however is not entirely switched off however, but the low level of activity that can be detected, and occasional bursts of the sex hormones that occasionally happen do not seem to encourage sexual development or alter gender behaviour.

The tendency for girls to start puberty at an earlier age than boys arises as a result of the gonadotropins FSH and LH being more amenable to activation in girls. Much been studied and written about the outcome in such situations. Precocious pubertal development and growth are also associated with precocious emotional development and earlier initiation of adult-orientated behaviours such as drug taking, sexual intercourse, and disruptive behaviours. However, no alterations in gender identity have been reported in early developing girls. Delay in the onset of puberty is more common in boys than girls as a result of the physiological differences. Late developing boys do not exhibit any differences in gender behaviour patterns. On the contrary, there is usually heightened anxiety at the lack of adult male defining physical features.

At the average age of onset of puberty, which ranges between 8 and 13 years in girls and 9 and 14 years in boys, the rate at which children develop features of adolescence and hence adulthood runs as a different pattern between each of the sexes. It is well recognised that girls show the outward signs of puberty much earlier than boys, together with a growth spurt earlier in age usually around 12 years. They may complete their passage to sexual and reproductive maturity, the attainment of menarche or menstrual periods within 2 to 3 years of puberty onset, whereas with boys, the pace of testosterone secretion is very slow in the first year to 18 months, after which the pace accelerates as does the growth rate and then the appearance of secondary sexual characteristics. There is no equivalent of menarche in girls as a major reproductive landmark in male puberty. Sperm production occurs right from the start of puberty in boys, and the first ejaculation can occur at variable ages from mid-puberty onwards depending upon whether that is spontaneous or produced by physical stimulation.

The pattern of physical and emotional development in each of the sexes is remarkably constant, yet for trans and gender diverse adolescents, the extent of the reaction to the physical change and function and the timing of its onset can differ markedly between adolescents irrespective of their birth assigned gender. In gender-non-conforming adolescents who were registered female at birth, this can range from a mild dislike of breast development and the menstruation-associated emotional lability to an extreme disquiet of the extent to which it is impossible to discuss the process. Others may exhibit a tolerance of their physical body, yet retain a more masculine outlook enhanced by clothing, hairstyles, and voice management. However, only a minority clearly express the desire to identify as non-binary when referred to consider any potential interventions.

The early physical and emotional changes of puberty are often not noticed in birth assigned males, but the mid-pubertal acceleration phase associated with height and weight gain and body shape changes from around 13 years of age signal that puberty is happening. It may be voice deepening which triggers gender dysphoria, whereas others are able to tolerate these physical changes and body or facial hair is the main concern. Functional reminders of the birth assigned gender such as the occurrence of erections and ejaculation can be the source of the disquiet, whereas sexuality and sexual function linked to their birth assigned gender may be tolerated and even enjoyed by some young people with gender dysphoria who detest the other physical changes such as body or facial hair. However, despite an extreme loathing of male functioning in some, it is usual to be able to have a discussion about semen preservation and how this is achieved without encompassing a major negative reaction if the topic is introduced by encouraging the young person to think about the future, and whether they might wish to create a home environment with their life partner, and whether they might think about taking steps to having a biologically related family of their own. Semen preservation is something that can be more readily entertained or even tolerated by those who have already begun masturbation or mutual sexual exploration. Indeed with techniques as they stand at present, physical stimulation in a birth assigned male is the only possible method to achieve this, and the young person needs to have developed at least mid-way through puberty.

One major challenge in knowing what an individual's ultimate position on the gender identification spectrum is going to be is when they haven't experienced the effects of sex hormones produced by their own sex glands. Although the maturation process begins at the onset of puberty, the extent to which any dysphoria may be expressed does not necessarily seem to depend on the extent to which the changes of puberty have developed. Whereas classically with the most extreme forms of dysphoria, trans men would be seeking breast removal and surgical augmentation of the genitalia and trans women would seek genital reconstructive surgery, with the larger numbers of adolescents presenting to the gender identity development service it would seem, within the current cohort, that the degree of dysphoria is less polarised, perhaps more fluid, and a willingness to accept non-binary or indeed mixed-gendered patterns is growing.

There does, however, seem to be more polarisation of gender around breast development. Many younger trans adolescents who were birth assigned female feel strongly that the breasts are the cardinal focus of their dysphoria and wish for an early mastectomy, whereas fewer are as strongly determined to have genital reassignment early on in the process, thinking this is a decision for the longer term. Birth assigned males are usually very keen to acquire oestrogen-derived breast development in order to satisfy personal and external female identification.

In birth assigned males, the primary objective of any intervention is to halt major virilizing effects, particularly voice lowering, Adam's apple development, facial and body hair, square jaw line, and muscle growth, all of which are a source of distress. In general, these factors generate anxiety to a much greater extent than concerns about the presence of male genitalia and their function.

Although hoped for by many on the embarkation of treatment, the GnRH analogue may not cause complete suppression of erectile function. Penile erection is primarily a neuro-vascular effect, enhanced by a sex hormone-dependent libido. In mid-adolescent birth-assigned males who have already embarked upon physical and sexual relationships, suppression of erectile function is not usually complete; Indeed, this partial effect may be beneficial as variability of sexuality, and a tolerance of both male and female anatomy, may eventually develop.

Paradoxically, despite increasing numbers of young people with dysphoria being referred to gender identity services, it would seem that there is a more of a gender ambivalence overall. However, early initiation of puberty blockade may actually lead to alterations in the long-term gender status, preventing maturation of physical body tolerance and normal adolescent sexual self and mutual experimentation. This intervention in itself may therefore not allow a non-binary status to develop over time.

Endocrine Manipulation of Sexual Development and Function

The use of the GnRH analogues to provide competitive blockade and consequent shutdown of the reproductive hormone system is well understood. It is a more complex process in adolescents than in adulthood as the hormone production process is working in overdrive at that time. The same treatment used for testosterone suppression in adult men with prostate cancer and to suppress oestradiol in women with endometriosis is consequently much easier to manage. The reproductive axis is actually rarely completely switched off in trans adolescents, but adequate sex hormone suppression is usually achieved in order to allow further psychosocial examination of their gender identity development.

Other commonly used anti-androgens such as cyproterone acetate and spironolactone (generally in adults) only provide partial hormone suppression and therefore an incomplete gonadal arrest and are probably too ineffective to be considered as suitable treatment for those adolescents with extreme dysphoria. However, in birth-assigned males, they can reduce some features of dysphoria such as hair growth and erectile function.

In birth-assigned females who have been through menarche, halting of menstruation alone may provide significant relief from the dysphoria and aid gender exploration. Standard-dose combined oral contraceptive pills (incorporating an oestrogen and a progestogen) when taken continuously without a break are useful to stop menstruation occurring. In this situation, it is generally recommended to have a planned withdrawal bleed once or twice a year for gynaecological health. However, the addition of an oestrogen, often misconceived as a female-only hormone, may contribute to worsening of the dysphoria as this treatment may continue to promote female physical development and breast growth. Oral progestogens such as norethisterone can provide instant and usually successful relief from menstruation for the short- to medium term during gender exploration. They need to be taken 2 to 3 times daily, so remembering to take the medication is key. Injectable depot preparations of progestogens, such as depot medroxyprogesterone acetate, are usually only partially successful in suppressing menstruation. However, they, as well as the combined oral contraceptive pill, are designed to be effective as contraceptives in those wishing to have vaginal intercourse. Progestogen containing intrauterine implants (coils) may provide longer-term (up to five years) suppression of menstruation and provide contraception too in those in whom gender dysphoria centres around the menstrual bleed.

None of the anti-androgenic preparations, including the GnRH analogue, can be sufficiently relied on in birth-assigned males to retain erectile function during sexual activity, and cannot be considered as satisfactory male contraceptives either.

In non-binary individuals, it may be theoretically possible to use a combination of the above therapies to reduce or halt the aspects of the physical bodily functioning which are exacerbating the dysphoria.

Current cross-sex hormone treatments are intended to induce the full range of physical secondary sex characteristics associated with the desired sex. In current practice, most adolescent gender identity centres follow standard incremental sex hormone treatment regimens similar to those used for the induction of pubertal characteristics in cisgender[1] adolescents over approximately 2 years. The main types of treatments used in trans men are injectable testosterone esters or transdermal testosterone gel; and in trans women, either oral oestradiol or transdermal oestrogen patches.

Some non-binary young people may wish to transition along the same pathway as fully identifying young trans men or women, whereas others may consider acquiring some features of the 'opposite' birth gender, but not develop the full set, retaining some of their birth-gender sex characteristics. This is an area where little experience has been gained at the present time in adolescents to give any indication of outcome. Theoretically, it could be possible to achieve a bespoke non-binary-appearing body using different schedules of sex hormone treatment producing partial sex-hormone-dependent changes; however, secondary sex characteristics once acquired are irreversible on stopping an unwanted sex hormone. Additionally, the sequence of acquisition of secondary sex characteristics when cross-sex hormone treatment is given is the same as naturally occurring puberty. This sequence can be stopped on withdrawal of the relevant hormone, but it is not possible to pick and choose specific characteristics without others which would normally occur concurrently.

External Factors Which Influence Non-binary Gender Identification

Young people presenting post-pubertally will have had experience of birth assigned sex hormone-driven development and function. Despite this, an element of choice and tolerance can be expressed in those whose gender identity falls towards the middle of the classic spectrum irrespective of the extent of sex hormone exposure. It appears that a middle ground may become more common and widely accepted.

For those whose gender dysphoria began at a very young age and who have changed their social role to that of the 'opposite' gender, the likelihood of finding a more non-binary identity/expression may be more difficult on account of having already made a polarity switch within the binary system. This can also be made more challenging by the family and external environment in their drive to fully support their child by facilitating the transition and subsequently reinforcing it by the strength of their support. The young person may lack either the courage or the confidence to change family, social, and school circles for a second occasion, and a non-binary status is less culturally understandable and possibly less tolerated than the transgender binary situation.

Blockade of puberty at the earliest possible time permissible, currently in early puberty (Tanner stage 2), may actually result in starting treatment at quite a young age (for puberty stages, see Marshall & Tanner, 1969, 1970). The social and emotional maturity of individuals as young as 9 or 10 years of age is significantly different from that of 16- or 17-year-olds. Knowledge of sex, reproduction, and fertility is distant and theoretical rather than lived-out, and is talked-about concepts rather than personal ones. The capacity for informed consent may well be questionable in very young adolescents and those with learning difficulties. The young person needs to be able to understand the benefits and complexities of a choice to start or not to start puberty blockade. In reality, this concept may not be fully understood until they are much older.

Current hormone treatment programmes in early-onset gender dysphoria include the GnRH analogue to suppress all cisgender secondary sex characteristic development. The young person therefore remains in a state of arrested puberty and also most probably with a form of arrested emotional development until cross-sex hormone treatment is considered suitable. Cross-sex hormone regimens are similar to those used in inducing the full range of pubertal changes in cisgender individuals, but are usually taken at a slower pace as the young person will have had minimal exposure to endogenous sex hormone production. It is notable that in the principal Dutch study of the outcome in young people starting GnRH analogue blockade at the onset of puberty, none has reportedly changed their mind about persisting with their full transgender status, and none has as yet taken a non-binary route (de Vries et al., 2014).

There is a risk, therefore, that we are seeing a newer group of young people entering adolescence and young adult life who have been exposed to a much more rigid endocrine manipulation pathway and paradoxically therefore are less likely to have the chance of expressing a non-binary gender than those going through a spontaneous puberty and experiencing the full effect of mature levels of their own spontaneously produced sex hormones. Although in a post-pubertal individual it is possible to "tinker round the edges" by part-oestrogenizing a birth-assigned-male with oestradiol, or part-virilizing a birth-assigned female with testosterone, this is not possible in those undergoing sex hormone blockade from the start of puberty as they will require full-dose cross-sex hormone replacement in due course for their general health and well-being—including energy, sexual function, and bone health. The attempt at producing a non-binary sex hormone environment would indeed not just be endocrinologically challenging, but also ethically worrying, as any attempt to provide a very low level hormone replacement regimen to align with gender preferences may possibly be inadequate for normal health, so paradoxically, non-binary gender identity may be a form of gender identity expression which would be less prevalent in the early-onset, early-blocked young people purely on account of the hormone treatment schedules.

Much additional research and long-term follow-up is required, particularly in the new wave of young people presenting de novo with much greater gender fluidity and non-binary expression.

Summary

- Human sex development is on a binary pattern.
- Diversity/Disorder/Differences of sex development rarely produce a non-binary gender.
- The presentation of non-binary gender status in adolescents does not seem to relate to the age of puberty onset.
- Extreme gender dysphoria during puberty is rare, with increasing numbers of teenagers exhibiting non-binary elements.
- Certain elements of pubertal development such as menstruation can be halted without the need for other major hormonal reversal.
- Early puberty blockade may fix the dysphoria and not permit the development of a fluid, non-binary gender expression.

Note

1. A cisgender person is a person content to remain the gender they were assigned at birth.

References

de Vries, A. L. C., McGuire, J. K., Steensma, T. D., Wagenaar, E. C. F., Theo, A. H., Doreleijers, T. A. H., et al. (2014). Young Adult Psychological Outcome After Puberty Suppression and Gender Reassignment. *Pediatrics, 134*(4), 696–704.

Marshall, W. A., & Tanner, J. M. (1969). Variations in Pattern of Pubertal Changes in Girls. *Archives of Disease in Childhood, 44*(235), 291–303.

Marshall, W. A., & Tanner, J. M. (1970). Variations in the Pattern of Pubertal Changes in Boys. *Archives of Disease in Childhood, 45*(239), 13–23.

Further Reading

Butler, G. E., & Kirk, J. M. W. (2011). *Oxford Specialist Handbook of Paediatric Endocrinology and Diabetes.* Oxford: Oxford University Press.

Hembree, W. C., Cohen-Kettenis, P., Delemarre-van de Waal, H. A., Gooren, L. J., Meyer III, W. J., Spack, N. P., et al. (2009). Endocrine Treatment of Transsexual Persons: An Endocrine Society Clinical Practice Guideline. *Journal of Clinical Endocrinology & Metabolism, 94*(9), 3132–3154.

Meriggiola, M. C., & Gava, G. (2015b). Endocrine Care of Transpeople Part I. A Review of Cross-sex Hormonal Treatments, Outcomes and Adverse Effects in Transmen. *Clinical Endocrinology, 83*, 597–606.

Meriggiola, M. C., & Gava, G. (2015a). Endocrine Care of Transpeople Part II. A Review of Cross-Sex Hormonal Treatments, Outcomes and Adverse Effects in Transwomen. *Clinical Endocrinology, 83*, 607–615.

Rosenthal, S. M. (2014). Approach to the Patient: Transgender Youth: Endocrine Considerations. *Journal of Clinical Endocrinology & Metabolism, 99*, 4379–4389.

10

Adult Endocrinology

Leighton Seal

Introduction

This chapter briefly reviews the biological basis for gender identity development and discusses the implications for non-binary gender identity. There will be a description of the implications of hypogonadism on physical health concentrating on the impact of low sex steroid levels on bone health, cardiovascular risk, and general wellbeing.

In discussing the hormonal management of non-binary gender identity, we have to accept that there is no robust literature on this subject. We have to rely on what is known about the process of gender differentiation; puberty induction in cisgender individuals that fail to go through puberty normally; and the hormonal management of trans people who

L. Seal (✉)
Charing Cross Gender Identity Clinic,
London, UK

© The Author(s) 2017
C. Richards et al. (eds.), *Genderqueer and Non-Binary Genders*, Critical and Applied
Approaches in Sexuality, Gender and Identity, DOI 10.1057/978-1-137-51053-2_10

transition from one gender to another and who identify within the binary of male or female (whom we shall call trans men or trans women from now on).

Biological Theory of Gender Identity Development

The development of gender identity is a complex interplay of psychological, social, and physical influences resulting in an internal and external expression of gender. Within the biological models of brain gender development, it is recognised that there are differences in the anatomy of some neural structures between males and females (Seal, 2007; Swaab et al., 1993), and in animal models, these areas accumulate testosterone and aromatise this to oestradiol, which has profound effects on neural restructuring by programmed cell death (apoptosis) (Hutchison, 1997). It is recognised that in mammals, gender-specific behavioural patterns, such as sexual behaviour in rats, can be altered by the administration (Bloch & Mills, 1995; Bloch, Mills, & Gale, 1995) or ablation of testosterone (Diaz, Fleming, & Rhees, 1995; Rhees, Kirk, Sephton, & Lephart, 1997) during a critical window in development. Although the critical window in humans has not been established, we do know that there are two significant peaks in testosterone production in human male foetuses at 12- to 14-week gestation (Reyes, Boroditsky, Winter, & Faiman, 1974; Tapanainen, Kellokumpu-Lehtinen, Pelliniemi, & Huhtaniemi, 1981) and a second peak in the first 3 months postnatally (Forest, de Peretti, & Bertrand, 1980), which are presumed to have a role in setting neural apoptosis patterns later in neural development (Hutchison, 1997).

In trans people, the neuro-anatomy (Zhou, Hofman, Gooren, & Swaab, 1995) and functional studies of the brain (Simon et al., 2013) suggest that the anatomy, and possibly the function of the brain, in this situation is more reflective of the person's internal gender (experienced gender) as opposed to the phenotypic gender of their somatic and hormonal milieu.

In the case of non-binary gender identities, there are, however, at present no studies of the neurobiological function or structural studies of the brain.

Hormone Treatment for Non-binary Gender Identity

As there are no clearly established guidelines for the hormonal treatment of non-binary people, and a lack of empirical evidence on which to base practice, it is important that the treatment of an individual with physical measures such as hormone or surgical interventions is done in the context of a multidisciplinary team (MDT) where the aspirations of the individual with regard to the physical parameters that will express their gender outwardly can be explored extensively.

This exploration needs to be done in the context of psychological expression of the individual's personal gender identity and their expectations of the physical changes in their body that therapy will produce. It is important that a clear formulation of the ideal mix (or lack) of masculine and feminine physical features the individual desires is established. This will form the basis on which discussions around what is feasible, achievable, and safe with hormone therapies can start, so that an increased congruence between the internal sense of gender and the outward expression of this can be achieved. Both the therapist exploring gender and the endocrinologist should be aware of the limitations and expected outcomes of hormone therapies in order to allow accurate advice—and potentially supportive counselling (see Barker & Iantaffi, this volume)—to be given with the aim of establishing a treatment plan the clinician and client agree to be the most effective form of therapy for the individual.

Hormonal and Physical Changes in Puberty

The developmental changes in puberty, apart from the changes in gonadal size that are produced by increasing gonadotrophin production, are due to the effect of oestrogen or testosterone production. There is a set sequence of events that occur in both boys and girls as defined by Tanner and Marshall (Marshall & Tanner, 1969, 1970). When inducing the secondary sexual characteristics of the individual's experienced gender with cross-sex hormone therapy, the same pattern of changes occurs. This has important implications for those desiring some of the effects produced by sex steroid use, but not others. The physiology of puberty is therefore of great relevance to this.

Puberty of Natal Females

In natal females, the first stage of pubertal development is adrenal sex steroid production, adrenarche, which precedes the onset of breast development (thelarche) by approximately 2 years. Thelarche precedes the development of genital and axillary hair by several months and menarche (onset of menstruation) by 2 years. The stages of breast development begin with elevation of nipple only (stage 1), then a breast bud appears under the areola which enlarges (mean age 11.2 years, stage 2), following this breast tissue grows beyond areola but without contour separation (mean age 12.4 years, stage 3), next the areola-nipple complex projects above the breast tissue forming a secondary mound (mean age 13.1 years, stage 4), and finally adult breast contour (mean age 14.5 years, stage 5) (Marshall & Tanner, 1969). It is of note that breast development is complete by the onset of menstruation, which means that progesterone production is not important in the pubertal development of breast, as a female must ovulate to produce progesterone and breast development is complete by the time this occurs. Oestradiol levels in the circulation rise steadily during the first stages of puberty, but are still modest at 100 pmol/l by Tanner stage III, which is well within the normal range for a natal male, and 165 pmol/l by Tanner stage IV, which is the upper part of the natal male range (Swerdloff & Odell, 1975).

Physical Changes in Trans Women with Oestrogen Therapy

For trans women, breast development follows the pattern seen in female puberty above, with breast development initiating within 3 months of starting oestrogen treatment and being complete by 2 years (Hembree et al., 2009; Seal, 2015). As there is no literature on the development of other secondary sexual characteristics during puberty, such as hip development, facial softening, and the like, we need to look at the available literature on the use of hormones for gender transition in trans women.

The literature on hormonal treatment of trans women suggests that skin softening and female fat redistribution onset occurs early in the process (2–6 months), but is not complete for 2–3 years during which time the individual is exposed to an increasing oestrogen dose in most treatment regimens (Hembree et al., 2009).

Implications for Hormone Replacement in Non-binary People with a Male Phenotype Body

When advising non-binary people about the likely effects of hormone replacement, it is important to discuss which elements of the female secondary sexual characteristics they desire. Our knowledge of puberty and the physical changes seen with oestrogen therapy in trans women mean that even with modest exogenous oestrogen doses, significant breast development may occur. If breast development is not desired, it will be difficult to guarantee that no breast development will occur because the lowest oestrogen doses used can all induce breast development in some individuals. Unfortunately, it is difficult to predict the likely breast developed in any one individual as there is a wide variation in responses to hormone therapy.

The dermatological effects of oestrogen treatment occur quickly with skin softening and a reduction in the facial hair growth. Both facial and truncal hair shaft diameters decrease, and this effect is maximal after 4 months of treatment (Giltay & Gooren, 2000). However, beard area hair growth needs to be removed by physical measures (laser, electrolysis, or shaving) in the vast majority of cases (Seal, 2015). At low doses of oestrogen, it may be possible therefore to have facial skin softening, but female fat distribution would be unlikely.

It is also important to advise the individual about the likely side-effects of oestrogen therapy, which include a 20-fold increased risk of thromboembolic disease, hyperprolactinaemia, and gall stone development (van Kesteren, Asscheman, Megens, & Gooren, 1997).

Example 1

A 22-year-old Caucasian male-bodied person was born of a successful pregnancy following recurrent miscarriage. Puberty occurred at 12 years with gynaecomastia, and the physical phenotype was unremarkably male as an adult. They had an onset of anxiety, depression, and deliberate self-harm from 12 years of age. There was also a restricted eating pattern, with altered body image, but there was no formal diagnosis of anorexia nervosa made. In the late teenage years, panic attacks also were feature of their mental state and they used alcohol to excess in an attempt to control their feelings of unhappiness with their body.

With regard to their gender identity, they felt that they were neutrois and consulted a primary care gender specialist with regard to their gender feelings. Dysphoric feelings about their body were managed by a combination of Progynova 4 mg and spironolactone 200–300 mg. These medications reduced facial hair and body hair. They also suppressed erectile function, and this consolidated the individual's ideas of their gender-neutral gender identity. One year later, they underwent gender-neutralising surgery in the form of penectomy, orchidectomy, clitoroplasty; but no labioplasty nor vaginoplasty. They were referred for specialist endocrine input with regard to the ongoing management of their hormones. On discussion with them, they desired to maintain good general health, but did not want to have overtly female secondary sexual characteristics. They were pleased with the results of the genital surgery.

Clinical Issues

The issues faced by this individual were that significant breast growth had occurred to Tanner stage II with prominent breast buds bilaterally. They also wished to maintain a gender-neutral body outline rather than a female-type body fat distribution.

They were also suffering from a lack of energy and general drive, and their anxiety disorder was not stable or treated. With regard to bone health, they were osteopaenic at the spine (T-score of –2) and normal at the hip (with a T-score of –0.4), suggesting a pattern of bone mineral loss that was minor but present.

Management

The initial management, in view of the person's low bone mineral density (BMD), was an attempt to increase the plasma oestradiol level by using topical oestrogen gel (Sandrena 2 mg). As the person's oestrogen level increased, there was an increase in breast development, which led to a decrease in psychological functioning and the patient stopped eating. Over 3 months, there was a 7 kg weight loss and the body mass index fell to 16.5 kg/m².

The individual was finding it difficult to take sufficient oestrogen for bone health. Increasing breast development was psychologically difficult for them, and there was an increase in their anxiety disorder and a decrease in social functioning. They consequently wished to take low-dose oestrogen therefore to facilitate bone health, prevent menopausal hot flashes, and to improve general energy and drive. The hormonal therapy was changed to Progynova at 2 mg a day with testosterone gel 10 mg once per day. Vitamin D supplementation was commenced to improve bone mineralisation.

On this combination of therapies, breast development stabilised and the individual's anxiety decreased. Their eating pattern improved, and with a generalised increase in body weight, the breasts became less obvious, which improved the individual's self-image. The testosterone therapy increased the general energy and drive and did not alter libido. Repeat dual emission x-ray absorptiometry (DEXA) scanning 3 years later demonstrated improved BMD with a T-score of −1.2 at the lumbar spine.

Discussion

The combination of low-dose oestrogen and testosterone hormone replacement therapy in this individual has facilitated improvement in bone health and maintained their gender-neutral physical appearance. As discussed earlier in the chapter, testosterone in combination with oestrogen can improve BMD over oestrogen therapy alone (Watts et al., 1995) and, in this case, can provide the individual with a mix of male and female hormone exposure preventing an imbalance in the development of secondary sexual characteristics. The improved balance between male and female with regard to hormonal effects on affect is mirrored in this individual's improved internal sense of gender neutrality and subsequently an improvement in psychological functioning.

With regard to the pre-surgical management of the person, on reflection it may have been better if this individual had been treated with a combination of a gonadotrophin-releasing hormone analogue (GNRHa) or cyproterone acetate and low-dose oestrogen rather than spironolactone and a moderate oestrogen dose, which has resulted in significant breast development that was undesired by the individual.

Puberty in Natal Males

In natal males, the first stage of pubertal development is enlargement of the genitalia. The scrotal skin thins as the testes enlarge followed by enlargement of the penis. Pubic hair development starts about the same time as penile enlargement. The onset of body hair development commences within 6 months of pubic hair development (Tanner stage III) with the usual sequence being axillary hair, perianal hair, upper lip hair, preauricular hair, periareolar hair, and then beard area (Garibaldi & Chemaitilly, 2011; Marshall & Tanner, 1986). Arm, leg, chest, abdominal, and back hair darken over the next 2–4 years, but there is a wide variation in the final hair distribution of adult men. Some men do not develop full facial hair for up to 10 years after the completion of puberty (Garibaldi & Chemaitilly, 2011). When considering the voice breaking, this usually occurs between Tanner stages III and IV. This means that the development of body hair and voice breaking are occurring at the same time. It is therefore very difficult to have one of these processes occurring without the other, as the ambient testosterone levels are the same during both processes.

If we look at the changes in testosterone levels during puberty, we find that testosterone levels remain relatively low until advanced puberty. By Tanner stage III, the testosterone level is still around 4.3 nmol/l (Winter & Faiman, 1972), (with a range of 2.1–9.5 nmol/l (Hiort, 2002)), by Tanner stage IV 7.1 nmol/l (Winter & Faiman, 1972) with a range of 4.9–17.9 nmol/l (Hiort, 2002). Even when puberty is complete, the mean testosterone level is a modest 10.7 nmol/l (Winter & Faiman, 1972) but with a range of 11.1–29.9 nmol/l (Hiort, 2002). It is not until 18 to 19 years of age that final adult testosterone levels are achieved, which is long after gonadal puberty has finished (Swerdloff & Odell, 1975; Winter & Faiman, 1972). We know from androgen withdrawal studies that muscular strength and bulk is lost when testosterone levels are low and that testosterone replacement increases muscular bulk and strength (Wang et al., 2000). In cisgender men with testosterone levels below 10 nmol/l, there is an increase in muscular mass and a decrease in fat mass when testosterone is given to increase the plasma level above 14 nmol/l (Bhasin, 2003; Seal, 2009; Wang et al., 2000), and indeed supra-physiological testosterone replacement can increase this even further (Bhasin et al., 2005). These data suggest that testosterone levels need to be elevated to the normal range to achieve male pattern muscular development.

Physical Changes in Trans Men with Testosterone Therapy

The first changes experienced by trans men are genital, with the development of the clitoris and cessation of menses when testosterone therapy is introduced (Hembree et al., 2009; Seal, 2015). Increases in body hair and the deepening of the voice tend to occur within about 9–12 months of therapy, but body hair development is not complete for up to 5 years of testosterone treatment (Hembree et al., 2009; Seal, 2015). Scalp hair recession occurs at a testosterone level that is the same as that which induces body hair development, so it is not possible to achieve a male pattern of body hair growth without the occurrence of scalp hair thinning if the individual is genetically programmed to loose scalp hair in response to testosterone treatment. Testosterone therapy in trans men also results in an increase in lean body mass and upper body strength, with an accompanying decrease in body fat. As a result, there is an increase in muscle definition with a decrease in hip-to-waist ratio, which results in a more masculinised body shape (Meyer et al., 1981; Meyer et al., 1986). This onsets early in therapy at about 3–4 months, but again can take up to 5 years to complete (Hembree et al., 2009; Seal, 2015).

Implications for Hormone Replacement in Non-binary People with a Female Phenotype Body

The individual needs to be advised about the likely side-effects of testosterone therapy including the development of polycythaemia, dyslipidaemia, increased cardiovascular risk (which is still only one-third of that of the cisgender male population) (van Kesteren et al., 1997), and endometrial hyperplasia (Futterweit, 1998) which requires endometrial monitoring (Seal, 2015). The effects of testosterone on genital development mean that clitoral enlargement is an inevitable consequence of testosterone treatment (Meyer et al., 1986). Likewise, there is likely to be an increase in sexual drive as testosterone treatment that raised the testosterone to the upper part of the female normal range is known to increase libido in female-bodied individuals (Davis & Worsley, 2014).

Testosterone increases the growth of the larynx and this occurs at a stage of puberty where the testosterone level is still moderate (Winter & Faiman, 1972). If the individual desires masculinisation, but to not effect laryngeal growth, then very low doses of testosterone therapy will be needed, certainly below a plasma testosterone value of 7 nmol/l. In trans men, this effect usually appears after 6–12 months of testosterone therapy (Hembree et al., 2009). Hormone manipulation will not significantly affect the size of the breast or alter the body contour of the chest and consequently surgical intervention is required to achieve this if required. When considering the development of a masculine body fat distribution and physique, although the effect onsets early, in testosterone therapy (Hembree et al., 2009), it will take several years and is likely to require doses of testosterone that are well within the adult male range. Consequently, it would be unlikely to achieve somatic masculinisation without hirsutism and male pattern capital hair loss in susceptible individuals.

Testosterone does have effects on mood with increased social activation, aggression, and sexual drive (Seal, 2009). In the studies using low-dose testosterone therapy for sexual dysfunction in cisgender females, summarised by Davis and Worsley (2014), there have been no reports of aggression or impulsivity in women treated with androgens. Neither has there been a significant rate of behavioural side-effects of androgen treatment reported in trans men treated with full testosterone replacement doses (van Kesteren et al., 1997), although arousability and risk behaviour have been reported to increase (Van Goozen, Cohen-Kettenis, Gooren, Frijda, & Van de Poll, 1995). Although behavioural shifts are to be expected, there are no studies examining the behavioural effects of testosterone therapy in non-binary gender identity. Therefore, individuals should be advised about the possible changes in cognition with regard to social arousability, aggression, and increase in libido as possible effects of testosterone treatment and that the effect of testosterone on these parameters is as yet unquantified in this client group.

When we are considering the provision of partial androgenisation in this situation, two approaches have traditionally been employed, either dose titration of the androgens to achieve a level of masculinisation that is not full; or to give androgen therapy for a period of time to induce some masculinisation and then stop or reduce the androgen dose after that.

Using androgens for a period of time and then halting therapy can be useful where features such as clitoral growth, minor increase in body hair, and voice breaking are desired. These events occur in a predictable time pattern with clitoral growth first at 3 months (Hembree et al., 2009), and voice breaking as well as the development of facial hair later at 9–12 months (Hembree et al., 2009). Over this time period, increase in muscular strength will happen and behavioural changes in arousability and libido will also happen. If full-dose androgen replacement is used to achieve masculinisation, then menses will stop.

On cessation of the androgen therapy, body hair patterns will regress to a female distribution, but if facial hair development has occurred, this is less likely to regress without local interventions such as laser and electrolysis. The body fat distribution and muscular strength will regress to a female pattern. Clitoral development is usually complete by 12 months, and clitoral growth is not likely to regress on stopping androgens. If the person is amenorrhoeic, then menstruation will return. To use this method of androgen treatment, there needs to be a clear understanding of the person's aims of treatment with regard to the degree of masculinisation they want, but also a thorough exploration of what the impact of a return of expressively female characteristics such as menstruation, reduced body hair, and female body composition will have on the individual after a period of masculinisation. The risk of this approach is that fluctuating hormone levels may cause a flair up of body dysphoria and the person will inevitably have periods of time when they are not in a steady state hormonally, which may lead to emotional liability.

The other approach is to use lower levels of androgen in the longer term. Here, we must aim to correlate the testosterone values seen in puberty (see section *puberty in natal males*) with the physical changes desired and not desired by the individual. This approach needs the individual to be fully aware of what is a likely outcome of their hormone therapy and indication of what is possible, that is, if facial hair development is desired, clitoral growth is inevitable. This approach has the disadvantage that higher doses of androgen are required for some feature of masculinisation such as changes in strength, but other features such as body hair increases occur at a lower threshold, so giving the ideal mix of feminine and masculine features may be difficult to achieve. It does however have the advantage of having steady hormone levels, which can allow for a more predictable effect on mood and emotional state.

Example 2

A 25-year-old female-bodied person was born by a normal vaginal delivery at term with normal childhood milestones. Puberty occurred early at the age of nine and menses settled down to a regular bleed 5 days every 28 days. Their gender dissonance onset at puberty and previous to this, they would wear their brother's underwear in primary school. Deliberate self-harm in the form of cutting of the upper part of the arm started from the age of 10 and went right the way through to the age of 16. Breast development was particularly difficult as it was felt to be a strong marker of a female gender. However, as they were sexually attracted to females they initially identified as a lesbian, but they soon realised that this description did not fit with their internal sense of self.

At university at the age of 21, they came into contact with trans people and at a trans youth support group were able to explore their gender identity more fully. They found that they definitely found female pronouns difficult; they were more accepting of male pronouns, but the best fit for them was to use gender-neutral pronouns. They therefore formulated their gender identity as being genderqueer. Their current partner is a female-bodied cisgender person who identifies their sexuality as queer.

Their past medical history was complicated by the presence of a microprolactinoma, but there was no suppression of the hypothalamo-pituitary-gonadal axis or other pituitary function.

They were assessed at a gender specialist clinic that referred for male chest reconstruction as they felt this was important in consolidating their genderqueer identity. Following the surgery, they felt that further masculinisation would be desirable to facilitate a non-female gender presentation.

Clinical Issues

The individual identifies as genderqueer and therefore does not want to have an overtly masculine appearance as they wish to be outside the gender binary and not to exchange one gender pole for another. They do not want the development of overtly masculine features to impact on their relationship with their partner. In addition, the therapy offered should not impact on the prolactinoma.

Management

After consideration by the MDT, the various forms of testosterone treatment were discussed and they were commenced on low-dose testosterone gel at half the dose usually used for cross-sex hormone therapy. They were commenced on calcium and vitamin D therapy, and DEXA scanning was arranged to ensure adequate bone mineralisation.

Outcome

On review, they found the increase in facial hair and body hair acceptable as they could control it by shaving. They found the masculinisation of facial features was positive as this meant that they were no longer perceived as female by strangers and the default pronouns used by people they did not know were male which was more acceptable to them than female pronouns. Menstruation continued but was acceptable to them. They now identify as a trans-masculine genderqueer person and use neutral gender pronouns amongst friends; but are accepting of male pronouns in the work environment or when interacting with people that do not know them.

They feel happy with their current gender expression and indeed their gender expression is more congruent with their gender identity. They do not want to increase the testosterone dose at present but feel this may be something they would like to explore in the future. There has been no increase in prolactin levels and BMD was normal.

Discussion

It has been important to establish with this person where they place themselves on the gender spectrum and also what the limits are with regard to progressing towards a masculine phenotype. With treatment, this person's gender identity has undergone a subtle shift towards masculinity as the initial stance of not wanting hormone treatment changed after male chest reconstruction and the person's view of the use of the term *male* to describe them changed after hormone therapy. It is important that the person's position on the gender spectrum be reviewed regularly as it may not be static and consequently decisions about increasing the dose of testosterone treatment should be done only after advising them regarding the likely increase in masculine secondary sexual characteristics that the person can expect; and the impact this would have on their non-binary gender identity. In this case, the physical health of the individual has not been impacted by hormone therapy, but again this needs regular review.

Gender-Neutralising Treatments

For some non-binary individuals, the aim of treatment is not to alter their secondary sexual characteristics but to neutralise them without developing the secondary sexual characteristics of another gender. This group of people may define themselves as *neuter*, *neutrois*, or *agender* among other terms. Hormonal therapy for this is possible using agents such as GnRHa that reduce the production of luteinising hormone (LH) and follicle-stimulating hormone (FSH) and hence gonadal sex steroid production.

Anti-androgens in male-bodied individuals; or progestins or the combined oral contraceptive pill in female-bodied individuals, can reduce the production of gonadal sex steroids, but they have hormone actions themselves—for example, Spironolactone can produce breast development and the oral contraceptive can promote female secondary sexual characteristics. Suppression of the reproductive axis makes the individual hypogonadal, and this will have metabolic and reproductive health consequences.

Implications of Hypogonadism and Hormone Therapy

Normal sex steroid levels are required for the maintenance of many systems in adult humans. Giving gender-neutralising therapy or sex steroid replacement at low doses can result in either no, or very low, production of the sex steroids in the body—making the individual either fully or partially hypogonadal. A review of hypogonadism itself is beyond the scope of this chapter, but the main systems that are affected by a lack of sex steroids are the cardiovascular system, musculoskeletal system, and reproductive systems.

Cardiovascular Health

In natal females, oestradiol deficiency results in an increased risk of cardiovascular disease (CVD). This occurs physiologically after menopause and is primarily due to alterations in lipid metabolism such that there is an increase in LDL cholesterol with a concomitant decrease in HDL cholesterol (Kannel, 2002; Lee & Foody, 2008). However, there is also an increase in triglycerides after menopause (Lee & Foody, 2008). These parameters improve with oestrogen therapy in post-menopausal women (Hale & Shufelt, 2015). The effects of oestrogen therapy on cardiovascular risk have been a topic of hot debate in the endocrine literature, with the original increase in cardiovascular events (stroke 1.14 [95% confidence interval (CI): 1.07–1.85]) and CVD event 1.29 [95% CI: 1.02–1.63] seen in the Women's Health Initiative trial resulting in the premature termination of the trial (Rossouw et al., 2002). This was followed by extensive sub-group analysis, which confirmed the excess in CVD was seen in those who initiated oestrogen more than 10 years post-menopause (Rossouw et al., 2007); whilst younger women had no excess cardiovascular risk. Further meta-analysis of 23 randomised controlled trials of women receiving HRT again demonstrated a 32% reduction in cardiovascular events (Salpeter, Walsh, Greyber, & Salpeter, 2006). These data suggest that, providing there is not a significant time without sex steroid exposure, oestrogen HRT can maintain cardiovascular health. Moreover, a recent study suggested that low-dose HRT has an equal effect on cardiovascular parameters to standard HRT doses (Matsui et al., 2014).

In trans women, there appears to be a slight increase in the standard mortality ratio (Asscheman et al., 2011; Dhejne et al., 2011), partly due to an increase in cardiovascular deaths (Asscheman et al., 2011). The increase in vascular disease appears to be associated with the current use of ethinyloestradiol, but not other oestrogen types (Asscheman et al., 2011), and so this oestrogen type is currently avoided in cross-sex hormone therapy regimens.

In natal males, hypogonadism is associated with an increase in CVD as there is a correlation between testosterone level and the incidence of coronary artery disease (Baulieu, 2002). Hypogonadal men also have other elements of metabolic syndrome including central obesity, reduced lean body mass, increased fat mass hypertension, and insulin resistance (Nieschlag & Behre, 2004). Testosterone replacement improves all of these parameters (Bhasin et al., 2006; Nieschlag & Behre, 2004), and the onset of these effects is within 90 days of initiation of treatment (Wang et al., 2000). In trans men, there is an alteration in the lipid profile of the individual so that there is a decrease in HDL and increase in LDL cholesterol and an increase in triglycerides (Mueller et al., 2010). The cardiovascular risk of trans men overall does not appear to increase with testosterone treatment and indeed the myocardial infarction risk of trans men is one-third that of cisgender males (Asscheman et al., 2011; van Kesteren et al., 1997). The overall standardised mortality ratio for trans men is 1 (Asscheman et al., 2011). This demonstrates that there is not an excess cardiovascular risk in the longer term with testosterone therapy for trans men, who use monitored standard cross-sex hormone replacement therapy.

Musculoskeletal System

Sex steroids are important in the maintenance of normal BMD in both males and females (Melmed & Williams, 2011), and consequently, hypogonadism in both sexes results in a reduction in BMD (Gambacciani & Ciaponi, 2000; Gambacciani et al., 1993; Melmed & Williams, 2011).

In natal females, hormone replacement therapy with oestrogen improves bone mineralisation (Gambacciani & Ciaponi, 2000; Wells et al., 2002), and indeed, there has been evidence over the last few years that ultra-low HRT using doses of oestradiol as low as 0.5 mg daily can be effective in maintaining bone health (Gambacciani et al., 2008), suggesting that minimal doses of oestrogen, far lower than are usually used in trans female HRT, may be effective. The addition of testosterone to oestrogen improves bone mineralisation over oestrogen-only HRT (Watts et al., 1995), which suggests that combined oestrogen androgen HRT may be an effective method of preserving BMD in individuals born with a female body.

In natal males, testosterone replacement improves bone mineralisation, but the existing evidence suggests a moderate effect (Bhasin et al., 2006; Tracz et al., 2006), and the effect of low-dose testosterone replacement on bone mineralisation is unknown. Oestrogen is known to have an important role in bone mineralisation, including the development of cortical bones in males (Vanderschueren et al., 2014), so one could speculate that oestrogen therapy could be used therapeutically to maintain bone mineralisation in a male-bodied individual.

When considering hormone replacement therapy in binary trans people, the general literature suggests that in trans women, BMD is preserved (Dittrich et al., 2005; Seal, 2015; van Kesteren, Lips, Gooren, Asscheman, & Megens, 1998); There has, however, been a study demonstrating that cross-sectional area of bone is reduced with oestrogen therapy in trans women compared to a natal male population (Lapauw et al., 2008). In trans men, standard dose testosterone therapy increases BMD cortical bone thickness and size (Lips, van Kesteren, Asscheman, & Gooren, 1996; Ruetsche, Kneubuehl, Birkhaeuser, & Lippuner, 2005; Van Caenegem et al., 2012). There has been one study which suggested a decrease in BMD, and interestingly, there was an inverse relationship between gonadotrophin concentration and bone mass suggesting that low sex steroid concentrations may result in low bone mineralisation in trans men (van Kesteren et al., 1998).

The implications of these data on hormone replacement use in people with non-binary gender identity are important, as there are no data on bone health for people using low-dose hormone replacement or sex steroid withdrawal. We can say with certainty that if androgen or oestrogen deprivation therapy is used, then there will be a reduction in bone mineralisation that would lead to an increase in the risk of fracture. In natal males, low-dose oestrogen in the presence of androgen withdrawal is likely to maintain BMD. In natal females, the protection of the skeleton from sex steroid withdrawal with lower-dose testosterone therapy is not as certain and may lead to a decrease in BMD. With the current lack of reliable data on bone health in non-binary people receiving hormone therapy, bone mineralisation should be monitored by DEXA scanning after 2 years of therapy, and if BMD cannot be maintained by the levels of sex steroid used to assist the gender presentation of the individual, further measures such as bisphosphonate therapy, selective oestrogen-receptor modulator (SERM), or anabolic agent treatment to maintain bone health may be required. Individuals should be advised about the possible need for these agents before commencing therapy.

Reproductive System

Regardless of gender, sex steroid therapy provides negative feedback to the hypothalamus, which then suppresses the production of gonadotrophins and inhibits reproductive function. This is the principal by which the combined oral contraceptive pill achieves contraception by inhibiting LH and FSH production and hence preventing ovulation (Melmed & Williams, 2011). In males, testosterone treatment has been used as a contraceptive, though this has not been seen in general use (World Health Organization Task Force on methods for the regulation of male fertility, 1990). Sex steroid therapy will therefore decrease reproductive function, but usually this effect is reversible if the sex steroids are discontinued. In binary trans people, standard cross-sex hormone therapy impairs reproductive function, and it is a good practice to discuss procedures to ameliorate this effect on reproduction, such as gamete storage, with all individuals so that fertility can be preserved if that is the individual's wish (de Roo et al., 2016; Richards & Seal, 2014).

Sex steroid administration has effects on the reproductive and associated organs, as well as on the ability to reproduce. With regard to breast health in binary trans people; there is only one large cohort study (n = 2307) which reported the incidence of breast cancer in trans women as 4.1 per 100,000 person-years (95% CI: 0.8–13.0) (Gooren, van Trotsenburg, Giltay, & van Diest, 2013)—a rate which is the same as the background rate of breast cancer in natal males. These data are reassuring as they suggest that oestrogen therapy does not increase breast cancer risk in trans women (Gooren et al., 2013). The same study also suggests that in trans men, the breast cancer risk is also that of the background risk of natal male breast cancer (Gooren et al., 2013). It is of note, however, that male chest reconstruction does leave a residuum of breast tissue, and trans men and non-binary people who have undergone the same kind of chest reconstruction should be encouraged to perform regular chest self-examination. Indeed, there have been five cases of breast cancer in trans men reported in the world literature thus far (Gooren, 2014).

Trans women have an extremely low prostate cancer risk. There have only been four cases reported in the literature so far (Seal, 2015). In a recent 30-year follow-up study, the incidence of prostate cancer was 0.04% (Gooren & Morgentaler, 2013), which is extremely low compared to the population incidence of prostate cancer in natal males (Sánchez-Chapado, Olmedilla, Cabeza, Donat, & Ruiz, 2003). These data are reassuring from the point of view of considering oestrogen exposure of the prostate on cancer risk; however, all the trans women in these studies were orchidectomised and so comment cannot be made on the effects of oestrogen on prostate safety in the context of higher testosterone levels.

In trans men, we know that exogenous testosterone therapy is associated with the development of a polycystic morphology in the ovary (Grynberg et al., 2010); however, ovarian cancer risk appears to be very low (Mueller & Gooren, 2008). With regard to uterine health, there is a theoretical risk of endometrial hyperplasia in trans men via aromatisation of testosterone to oestradiol. Indeed, a small study reported a 15% risk of endometrial hyperplasia in trans men (Futterweit, 1998). The clinical impression is, however, that this risk is very overstated and histological studies on hysterectomy specimens taken from trans men consistently demonstrate endometrial atrophy (Grynberg et al., 2010). Currently, clinical practice recommends that trans men on testosterone therapy have their endometrial thickness monitored by 2-yearly ultrasound scanning and that hysterectomy is considered after 2 years of testosterone therapy (Seal, 2015).

The effects of the above changes on the function of the female reproductive tract are largely unknown. There has only been one study reporting outcomes of pregnancy in trans men who have withdrawn from androgen (Light, Obedin-Maliver, Sevelius, & Kerns, 2014). In this study, 80% of trans men had a return of menstruation within 6 months of cessation of testosterone treatment, and their pregnancies were not different to trans men that had not used testosterone prior to conception (Light et al., 2014). There was however a higher than expected incidence of post-natal depression in trans men at 12% (Light et al., 2014).

Vasomotor Symptoms

Vasomotor symptoms occur in sex steroid withdrawal in both genders. In female-bodied individuals, menopausal sweats and flushes occur at a plasma oestradiol level of around 30 pmol/l, which is about one-third of the normal female luteal levels (Gast, Samsioe, Grobbee, Nilsson, & van der Schouw, 2010). In male-bodied individuals, these occur at a plasma testosterone level of 4.5–5 Nmol/l, which is approximately half to one-third of the bottom end of the normal range for testosterone measurements (Zitzmann, Faber, & Nieschlag, 2006). Sex steroid replacement can resolve these symptoms in any gender.

Cognition

It is known that low sex steroid levels are associated with low energy, lack of motivation, and poor general drive (Aversa & Morgentaler, 2015; Mueller, Grissom, & Dohanich, 2014; Wang et al., 2000; Woods & Mitchell, 2005). Low levels of sex steroids can be associated with depression in both males and females, and hormonal replacement with sex steroids can alleviate these symptoms (Khera, 2013; Morgan, Cook, Rapkin, & Leuchter, 2005; Onalan et al., 2005). Libido also is correlated with plasma testosterone levels in both genders, and hypogonadism is therefore associated with a reduced libido (Anastasiadis, Davis, Salomon, Burchardt, & Shabsigh, 2002; Aversa & Morgentaler, 2015). People requesting gender-neutralising treatments need to be counselled about these as likely effects of the treatment. General health measures such as maintaining good general health, nutrition, and exercise should be suggested to reduce the impact of the lowering of energy.

Implications for Hormone Replacement in Non-binary People

For most non-binary people, a dose of sex steroid replacement lower than that for trans people is requested to limit the development of the secondary sexual characteristics of the non-natal gender to those desired. The doses of oestrogen used in cisgender females for hormone replacement are typically two to five times lower than those used for hormone replacement in transgender individuals (Hembree et al., 2009; Seal, 2007, 2015). When treating patients with non-binary gender identity, it is often the case that the individual desires the minimal amount of hormone possible to maintain health and not unduly impact on the development of unwanted secondary sexual characteristics.

In male-bodied people, it is therefore reassuring that standard HRT (Salpeter et al., 2006) or even ultra-low doses of oestrogen (Matsui et al., 2014), which will have minimal impact on physical development, should still provide adequate cardiovascular protection. In a similar vein, both standard and ultra-low oestrogen therapy would be expected to protect bone health (Gambacciani et al., 2008; Gambacciani & Levancini, 2014). The impact on reproductive function would be expected to be reversible after oestrogen therapy is withdrawn. The effect on prostate health is unknown, but as diethylstilboestrol was a recognised treatment for prostate cancer historically, it would not be predicted to impact negatively on prostate health (Turo et al., 2014). Vasomotor symptoms usually resolve in 80% of women using standard HRT oestrogen doses (Sassarini & Lumsden, 2015) and in 60% of those using ultra-low HRT doses (Matsui et al., 2014); so low-dose oestrogen therapy may be effective in suppressing vasomotor symptoms in HRT for non-binary gender people.

In female-bodied individuals, we know that standard dose testosterone therapy does not negatively impact on cardiovascular health, either in the short term when trans men's risk of myocardial infarction is one-third of the general male population (van Kesteren et al., 1997) or in the longer term, where there is no impact on the incidence of CVD (van Kesteren et al., 1998). The use of low-dose testosterone treatment in non-binary individuals would therefore be predicted to have a lower impact than even this and would most likely have an even smaller impact on cardiovascular health. This view is supported by studies on androgen therapy for post-menopausal libido disturbance which suggest that low-dose topical testosterone therapy does not impact on cardiovascular parameters (Davis et al., 2008; Davis & Worsley, 2014). The effect of low-dose testosterone treatment on bone health is not as certain. As studies in trans men suggest that inadequate testosterone treatment may reduce BMD (van Kesteren et al., 1998), low-dose testosterone therapy would be predicted to result in a loss of BMD that may require salvage with additional agents. It would seem sensible in this situation for non-binary female-bodied individuals to take calcium and vitamin D supplements for bone protection.

GnRH Analogues

When given continuously, GnRH analogues result in the suppression of LH and FSH production by the pituitary gland as the GnRH receptors are down regulated and down regulation of the GnRH receptors on the pituitary cells occurs (tachyphylaxis)(Melmed & Williams, 2011). Sex steroid withdrawal with the use of GnRH analogues would be predicted to impact on the health of the individual. There will be an adverse effect on cardiovascular health, dyslipidaemia, vasomotor symptoms, reduced BMD, and inhibited reproductive function. If the individual wishes to have sex steroid withdrawal to reduce the effects of their natal gender hormone production, these issues will need to be addressed.

Anti-androgens

In male-bodied people, anti-androgens can be considered to reduce masculine features without administering female hormones. However, they are all associated with the development of significant side-effects. For example, Cyproterone acetate is a progesterone derivative—the use of which is associated with the development of gynaecomastia and galactorrhoea, which may not be desired by a non-binary person. The degree of gynaecomastia to be expected is very variable and so it is difficult to advise an individual on the likely effect of this drug on breast growth, but it occurs in 20% of people treated with Cyproterone acetate (Neumann & Kalmus, 1991). Cyproterone acetate use is associated with liver dysfunction (Frey & Aakvaag, 1981; Willemse et al., 1988), development of meningioma (Gil et al., 2011), and also depression (Barth, Cherry, Wojnarowska, & Dawber, 1991; Frey & Aakvaag, 1981; Seal et al., 2012). This final side-effect is of particular importance as depression commonly co-exists in individuals with gender non-conformity (Seal et al., 2012). Finasteride is a 5-alpha-reductase type-2 inhibitor that reduces the conversion of testosterone to the more active dihydrotestosterone. This is therefore a mild anti-androgen and has a similar range of side-effects as Cyproterone acetate (Altomare & Capella, 2002; Ciotta et al., 1995), but does not cause significant gynaecomastia in clinical practice.

Spironolactone, in contrast, is a steroidal potassium-sparing diuretic, whose main pharmacological action is to act as a mineralocorticoid receptor antagonist, but it is also an androgen-receptor partial antagonist as well as an oestrogen-receptor agonist. As such, in addition to blocking the androgen receptor, it also has a significant oestrogenic action. Significant gynaecomastia is a common side-effect of this drug and can result in pronounced breast development. Through its mineralocorticoid receptor antagonism, it can cause hyperkalaemia and renal impairment. There have also been reports of Spironolactone use being associated with upper gastrointestinal bleeding (Gulmez et al., 2008). This side-effect profile, especially its effect on breast growth, limits the effectiveness of this agent when reducing masculinisation in male-bodied non-binary-gendered people. It is important however to note that anti-androgen treatment is ineffective in suppressing facial hair growth in trans women, and that facial hair can only be controlled by local measures such as laser, electrolysis, or shaving (Seal, 2015).

Progestins and Continuous Oral Contraceptives for Menstrual Suppression

The occurrence of menstrual bleeding for a significant number of non-binary female-bodied people is a profound signifier of femininity that they wish to ablate. Menstrual suppression can be achieved with the use of progestins and medroxyprogesterone (Fraser, 1990) or norethisterone (Saarikoski, Yliskoski, & Penttilä, 1990) which have been used to delay menstruation in natal females. These preparations can produce reliable amenorrhoea as the doses used are higher then used for oral contraception and for a non-binary person have the advantage that they do not produce feminising physical changes in the body. Depot preparations have also been used, but they can result in prolonged irregular bleeding in up to 25% of users (Fraser, 1994). Indeed, the majority of people will have some irregular bleeding in the first year (Jacobstein & Polis, 2014). This is of concern when using these agents in non-binary people, as an unpredictable bleeding pattern can be more negative psychologically than a predictable bleed.

Intrauterine progestin delivery systems too are associated with irregular menstrual bleeding when first used in 5–15% of people but produce an amenorrhoea rate of 70% over 5 years (Inki, 2007). Longer-term continuous progestin use does not appear to be harmful for the endometrium (Jeppsson, Johansson, Ljungberg, & Sjöberg, 1977). There have been concerns that prolonged progestin only use can result in a reduction in bone mineralisation with more than 2 years of continuous use (Jacobstein & Polis, 2014).

One option is the use of oral contraceptives which are usually given in a cyclical pattern with a 1-week pill-free period every month to allow menstrual bleeding. There have been several studies looking at extended regimens that provide menstrual suppression, usually on a quarterly basis. There was effective suppression of menstrual bleeding and no evidence of endometrial hyperplasia in these studies (Anderson, Feldman, & Reape, 2008; Anderson et al., 2005). There have been extended studies using suppression for 163 days, and this regimen was not associated with significant endometrial growth as assessed by pelvic ultrasound scanning (Kwiecien, Edelman, Nichols, & Jensen, 2003). For non-binary people where menstruation produces feelings of dysphoria, but other secondary sexual characteristics associated with female gender are not perceived as undesirable by the person, this could be a useful method of menstrual suppression providing endometrial monitoring can be achieved by bi-annual uterine ultrasound scanning, as recommended for trans men on testosterone therapy (Futterweit, 1998; Seal, 2015). For non-binary female-bodied people however, the thought of taking a female hormone can be felt to be a reinforcement of their birth gender and for many it is therefore not a treatment option they desire.

Non-hormonal Interventions

If the individual wants to have suppression of sex steroid production, but does not desire hormone interventions, then the impact of hypogonadism can be mitigated by using various agents to improve the metabolic state of the hypogonadal individual.

The reduction in BMD can be mitigated by the use of calcium and vitamin D supplementation. If BMD does decrease despite this, then other agents such as bisphosphonates, SERMs, or bone anabolic agents such as sodium ranelate or teriparatide can be used (Gambacciani & Ciaponi, 2000). However, these agents are associated with various side-effects such as jaw bone necrosis, oesophageal cancer, and gastric ulcers with bisphosphonates (McGreevy & Williams, 2011) and thromboembolism with strontium ranelate (McGreevy & Williams, 2011). Also, the cardiovascular implications of hypogonadism can be addressed by statin treatment for dyslipidaemia and control of weight and blood pressure with appropriate health advice and medications. Additionally, vasomotor symptoms can be addressed using either SSRI treatment, such as venlafaxine (Carroll & Kelley, 2009; Ensrud et al., 2015; Loibl et al., 2007), or a central alpha-blocking agent such as clonidine (Laufer, Erlik, Meldrum, & Judd, 1982). Study evidence suggests that SSRI treatment is superior to clonidine in reducing hypogonadal hot flushes (Loibl et al., 2007).

An Approach to Clinical Management

When deciding what hormonal interventions are appropriate for the individual, it is essential that the decisions are made in the context of a multidisciplinary approach. It is important that the degree of fluidity of the person's current gender expression is assessed; a clear formulation of the mix of male, female, and neutral physical features is made; and that significant co-existing psychological issues are excluded or managed.

It is also important to advise the individual that none of the hormone regimens used in this field have been examined by randomised controlled clinical trials and that the available therapeutic options are largely based on extrapolation from hormone replacement therapy in cisgendered and binary transgendered people. Table 10.1 outlines the dose ranges of current preparations used in the UK for hormone replacement in cisgender and transgender individuals as a guide of hormone doses in general usage. The approach to hormone therapy also needs to be individualised. Indeed, hormonal therapy may not be appropriate in some individuals, for example, a female-bodied person who has dysphoria regarding the presence of breasts may require only surgical intervention.

For others, hormones can be used to reduce the physical features of their birth sex and may or may not induce the secondary characteristics of their non-birth sex. In those that desire gender neutrality, GnRH analogues provide a means by which sex steroid production can be halted and reduce the effects of these hormones in the body. The resulting hypogonadism can be controlled by tailored hormone replacement with either low-dose natal sex hormone replacement, cross-sex hormone replacement, or a combination hormone replacement regimen. If sex steroid replacement is not desired, then non-hormonal interventions can be employed to reverse the effects of the induced hypogonadism. This approach has the advantage of having some predictability with regard to likely physical changes induced by the hormones at the doses being used. The disadvantage is that if the hormones are used at lower than usual doses used for cross-sex hormone replacement, then relative hypogonadism can occur and this must be monitored for any impact on physical health such as reduced BMD or increased cardiovascular risk which would need to be treated.

Table 10.1 A comparison of sex steroid doses in adult and paediatric cisgendered hormone replacement versus hormone replacement in transgendered individuals

Preparation	Binary trans female dose	Podiatric practice cisgender female dose	Adult cisgender female dose	Adult cisgender male dose
Oestradiol valerate: Or Oestradiol hemihydrate	1–8 mg daily	5–10 mcg/kg o.d	0.5–2 mg daily	–
Patches: Oestradiol	50–200 mcg/24 hr twice weekly	3.1–18.8 mcg/24 hr twice a week	25–100 mcg/24 hr twice a week	–
Topical Gel:	0.5–5 mg 1 mg sachets	–	0.5–2 mg daily	–
Ethinyloestradiol**	50–100 mcg daily	1–10 mcg daily	20–30 mcg (as combined oral contraceptive pill)	Diethylstilboestrol 1–2 mg daily for prostate cancer
Conjugated equine oestrogens **	1.25–5 mg daily	–	0.265–1.2 mg daily	–
Implants Oestrogen Implant	50–150 mg 6–24 monthly	–	50–100 mg 6–24 monthly	–
Preparation	Binary trans male dose	Paediatric practice cisgender male dose	Adult cisgender male dose	Adult cisgender female dose
Testosterone injections (monthly)	250 mgs Injection 4, 3, or 2 weekly (dose can be from 150 to 250 mgs)	25–50 mg weekly	250 mgs Injection 4, 3, or 2 weekly (dose can be from 150 to 250 mgs)	–
Longer acting testosterone injection	1000 mg 10–15 weekly	–	1000 mg 10–15 weekly	–
Topical testosterone gel	50 mg/5 gm daily	–	50 mg/5 gm daily	5 mg/0.5 ml daily

**Neither ethinyl estradiol or conjugated equine estrogens are commonly used as oestrogens in cross sex hormone therapy in the UK

The other approach is to allow natal hormone production to continue and attempt to suppress this sufficiently with anti-androgen therapy in a male-bodied person, or progestin or combined oestrogen/progestin treatment in a female-bodied person. This approach has the advantage that the induced hypogonadism may not be as profound as with GnRH analogues, but these agents will produce variable and difficult to quantify changes in the secondary sexual characteristics of the individual. For example, anti-androgens result in the development of gynaecomastia and may have other significant side-effects such as depression, hyperprolactinaemia, and GI bleeding, whereas progestins can result in unpredictable menstrual bleeding pattern before they inhibit menstruation.

In all people, it is important to discuss the fact that hormone therapy will impact on reproductive potential and that hormone therapies used in this way have an unquantified effect on reproductive function. In those that are female-bodied, it is important to discuss contraceptive issues as lower-dose hormone regimens may not suppress ovulation, but are likely to be teratogenic.

It is also good practice for the individual to be reviewed regularly by the members of the MDT so that the cadence of the physical changes can be assessed, the likely speed of progression to the development of further secondary sexual reviewed, and decisions about reversal of undesired changes in the body of the individual can be discussed.

Finally, it is important to have psychological input to the care of the individual, as the impact of the physical changes in the person on the psychological function, levels of dysphoria, and ongoing expectations of hormone therapy's effect on their gender presentation must be assessed to allow for an integrated programme of care to be delivered to the person.

Summary

There is no current literature on the hormonal management of people with a non-binary or neutrois gender identity. We therefore have to use physiological principals and literature on hormone replacement in trans people to guide our treatment decisions.

- Good clinical practice is to undertake hormone therapy decisions as part of an MDT where the aspirations of the individual with regard to the physical parameters that will express their gender outwardly can be explored fully.
- It is important that the degree of fluidity of the person's current gender expression is assessed; a clear formulation of the mix of male, female, and neutral physical features is made; and that significant co-existing psychological issues are excluded or managed.
- Both the therapist exploring gender and the endocrinologist should be aware of the limitations and expected outcomes of hormone therapies in order to allow accurate advice.
- Recommendations should be based on what is feasible, achievable, and safe with hormone therapies.
- The aim of treatment is an agreed regimen between clinician and client that results in an increased congruence between the internal sense of gender and the outward expression.

Implications of Hormone Replacement in Non-binary People with a Male Phenotype Body

- It will be difficult to guarantee that no breast development will occur because the lowest oestrogen doses used can all induce breast development in some individuals.
- The dermatological effects of oestrogen treatment occur quickly with skin softening and a reduction in the facial hair growth. However, beard area hair growth needs to be removed by physical measures (laser, electrolysis, or shaving).
- At low doses of oestrogen, it may be possible therefore to have facial skin softening, but female fat distribution would be unlikely.
- It is also important to advise the individual about the likely side-effects of oestrogen therapy, which include a 20-fold increased risk of thromboembolic disease, hyperprolactinaemia, and gall stone development.

Implications of Hormone Replacement in Non-binary People with a Female Phenotype Body

- The individual needs to be advised about the likely side-effects of testosterone therapy including the development of polycythaemia, dyslipidaemia, increased cardiovascular risk and endometrial hyperplasia which requires endometrial monitoring.
- The effects of testosterone on genital development mean that clitoral enlargement is an inevitable consequence of testosterone treatment.
- There is likely to be an increase in sexual drive with testosterone treatment.
- Testosterone increases the growth of the larynx, and this occurs at a stage of puberty where the testosterone level is still moderate.
- Hormone manipulation will not significantly affect the size of the breast or alter the body contour of the chest and consequently surgical intervention is required to achieve this if required.
- Somatic masculinisation requires doses of testosterone that are well within the adult male range and so will not occur without hirsutism and male pattern capital hair loss in susceptible individuals.
- Testosterone's effects on mood with increased social activation, aggression, and sexual drive appear to be dose dependent; but the effect of testosterone on these parameters is as yet unquantified in this client group.

Gender-Neutralising Treatments

- These will result in hypogonadism whose main effects are on the cardiovascular system, musculoskeletal system, cognition and reproductive systems.
- The resulting hypogonadism can be controlled by tailored hormone replacement with either low-dose natal sex hormone replacement, cross-sex hormone replacement, or a combination hormone replacement regimen. If sex steroid replacement is not desired, then non-hormonal interventions can be employed to reverse the effects of the induced hypogonadism.

References

Altomare, G., & Capella, G. L. (2002). Depression Circumstantially Related to the Administration of Finasteride for Androgenetic Alopecia. *The Journal of Dermatology, 29*(10), 665–669.

Anastasiadis, A. G., Davis, A. R., Salomon, L., Burchardt, M., & Shabsigh, R. (2002). Hormonal Factors in Female Sexual Dysfunction. *Current Opinion in Urology, 12*(6), 503–507. doi:10.1097/01.mou.0000039451.39928.49.

Anderson, F. D., Feldman, R., & Reape, K. Z. (2008). Endometrial Effects of a 91-day Extended-regimen Oral Contraceptive with Low-Dose Estrogen in Place of Placebo. *Contraception, 77*(2), 91–96. doi:10.1016/j.contraception.2007.11.006.

Anderson, F. D., Hait, H., Hsiu, J., Thompson-Graves, A. L., Wilborn, W. H., & Williams, R. F. (2005). Endometrial Microstructure After Long-term Use of a 91-Day Extended-cycle oral Contraceptive Regimen. *Contraception, 71*(1), 55–59. doi:10.1016/j.contraception.2004.07.013.

Asscheman, H., Giltay, E. J., Megens, J. A., de Ronde, W. P., van Trotsenburg, M. A., & Gooren, L. J. (2011). A Long-term Follow-Up Study of Mortality in Transsexuals Receiving Treatment with CROSS-sex Hormones. *European Journal of Endocrinology, 164*(4), 635–642. doi:10.1530/EJE-10-1038.

Aversa, A., & Morgentaler, A. (2015). The Practical Management of Testosterone Deficiency in men. *Nature Reviews Urology, 12*(11), 641–650. doi:10.1038/nrurol.2015.238.

Barth, J. H., Cherry, C. A., Wojnarowska, F., & Dawber, R. P. (1991). Cyproterone Acetate for Severe Hirsutism: Results of a Double-Blind Dose-Ranging Study. *Clinical Endocrinology, 35*(1), 5–10.

Baulieu, E. E. (2002). Androgens and Aging Men. *Molecular and Cellular Endocrinology, 198*(1–2), 41–49.

Bhasin, S. (2003). Effects of Testosterone Administration on Fat Distribution, Insulin Sensitivity, and Atherosclerosis Progression. *Clinical Infectious Diseases, 37*(Suppl. 2), S142–S149. doi:10.1086/375878.

Bhasin, S., Woodhouse, L., Casaburi, R., Singh, A. B., Mac, R. P., Lee, M., et al. (2005). Older Men are as Responsive as Young Men to the Anabolic Effects Of Graded Doses of Testosterone on the Skeletal Muscle. *The Journal of Clinical Endocrinology and Metabolism, 90*(2), 678–688. doi:10.1210/jc.2004-1184.

Bhasin, S., Cunningham, G. R., Hayes, F. J., Matsumoto, A. M., Snyder, P. J., Swerdloff, R. S., et al. (2006). Testosterone Therapy in Adult Men with

Androgen Deficiency Syndromes: An Endocrine Society Clinical Practice Guideline. *The Journal of Clinical Endocrinology and Metabolism, 91*(6), 1995–2010. doi:10.1210/jc.2005-2847.

Bloch, G. J., & Mills, R. (1995). Prepubertal Testosterone Treatment of Neonatally Gonadectomized Male Rats: Defeminization and Masculinization of Behavioral And Endocrine Function in Adulthood. *Neuroscience and Biobehavioral Reviews, 19*(2), 187–200.

Bloch, G. J., Mills, R., & Gale, S. (1995). Prepubertal Testosterone Treatment of Female Rats: Defeminization of Behavioral and Endocrine Function in Adulthood. *Neuroscience and Biobehavioral Reviews, 19*(2), 177–186.

Carroll, D. G., & Kelley, K. W. (2009). Use of Antidepressants for Management of Hot Flashes. *Pharmacotherapy, 29*(11), 1357–1374. doi:10.1592/phco.29.11.1357.

Ciotta, L., Cianci, A., Calogero, A. E., Palumbo, M. A., Marletta, E., Sciuto, A., et al. (1995). Clinical and Endocrine Effects of Finasteride, a 5 Alpha-reductase Inhibitor, in Women with Idiopathic Hirsutism. *Fertility and Sterility, 64*(2), 299–306.

de Roo, C., Tilleman, K., T'Sjoen, G., & de Sutter, P. (2016). Fertility Options in Transgender People. *International Review of Psychiatry, 28*(1), 112–119.

Davis, S. R., Moreau, M., Kroll, R., Bouchard, C., Panay, N., Gass, M., et al. (2008). Testosterone for Low Libido in Postmenopausal Women not Taking Estrogen. *The New England Journal of Medicine, 359*(19), 2005–2017. doi:10.1056/NEJMoa0707302.

Davis, S. R., & Worsley, R. (2014). Androgen Treatment of Postmenopausal Women. *The Journal of Steroid Biochemistry and Molecular Biology, 142*, 107–114. doi:10.1016/j.jsbmb.2013.05.006.

Dhejne, C., Lichtenstein, P., Boman, M., Johansson, A. L., Långström, N., & Landén, M. (2011). Long-Term Follow-Up of Transsexual Persons Undergoing Sex Reassignment Surgery: Cohort Study In Sweden. *PLoS One, 6*(2), e16885. doi:10.1371/journal.pone.0016885.

Diaz, D. R., Fleming, D. E., & Rhees, R. W. (1995). The Hormone-Sensitive Early Postnatal Periods for Sexual Differentiation of Feminine Behavior and Luteinizing Hormone Secretion in Male and Female Rats. *Brain Research. Developmental Brain Research, 86*(1–2), 227–232.

Dittrich, R., Binder, H., Cupisti, S., Hoffmann, I., Beckmann, M. W., & Mueller, A. (2005). Endocrine Treatment of Male-To-Female Transsexuals Using Gonadotropin-Releasing Hormone Agonist. *Experimental and Clinical Endocrinology & Diabetes, 113*(10), 586–592. doi:10.1055/s-2005-865900.

Ensrud, K. E., Guthrie, K. A., Hohensee, C., Caan, B., Carpenter, J. S., Freeman, E. W., et al. (2015). Effects of Estradiol and Venlafaxine on Insomnia Symptoms and Sleep Quality in Women with Hot Flashes. *Sleep, 38*(1), 97–108. doi:10.5665/sleep.4332.

Forest, M. G., de Peretti, E., & Bertrand, J. (1980). Testicular and Adrenal Androgens and Their Binding to Plasma Proteins in the Perinatal Period: Developmental Patterns of Plasma Testosterone, 4-androstenedione, Dehydroepiandrosterone and its Sulfate in Premature and Small for Date Infants as Compared with that of Full-Term Infants. *Journal of Steroid Biochemistry, 12*, 25–36.

Fraser, I. S. (1990). Treatment of Ovulatory and Anovulatory Dysfunctional Uterine Bleeding with Oral Progestogens. *The Australian & New Zealand Journal of Obstetrics & Gynaecology, 30*(4), 353–356.

Fraser, I. S. (1994). Vaginal Bleeding Patterns in Women Using Once-A-Month Injectable Contraceptives. *Contraception, 49*(4), 399–420.

Frey, H., & Aakvaag, A. (1981). The Treatment of Essential Hirsutism in Women with Cyproterone Acetate and Ethinyl Estradiol. Clinical and Endocrine Effects in 10 Cases. *Acta Obstetricia et Gynecologica Scandinavica, 60*(3), 295–300.

Futterweit, W. (1998). Endocrine Therapy of Transsexualism and Potential Complications of Long-Term Treatment. *Archives of Sexual Behavior, 27*(2), 209–226.

Gambacciani, M., Cappagli, B., Ciaponi, M., Pepe, A., Vacca, F., & Genazzani, A. R. (2008). Ultra Low-Dose Hormone Replacement Therapy and Bone Protection in Postmenopausal Women. *Maturitas, 59*(1), 2–6. doi:10.1016/j.maturitas.2007.10.007.

Gambacciani, M., & Ciaponi, M. (2000). Postmenopausal Osteoporosis Management. *Current Opinion in Obstetrics & Gynecology, 12*(3), 189–197.

Gambacciani, M., & Levancini, M. (2014). Hormone Replacement Therapy and the Prevention of Postmenopausal Osteoporosis. *Przeglad Menopauzalny, 13*(4), 213–220. doi:10.5114/pm.2014.44996.

Gambacciani, M., Spinetti, A., de Simone, L., Cappagli, B., Maffei, S., Taponeco, F., et al. (1993). The Relative Contributions Of Menopause and Aging to Postmenopausal Vertebral Osteopenia. *The Journal of Clinical Endocrinology and Metabolism, 77*(5), 1148–1151. doi:10.1210/jcem.77.5.8077305.

Garibaldi, L., & Chemaitilly, W. (2011). Physiology of Puberty. In R. Kliegman & W. E. Nelson (Eds.), *Nelson Textbook of Pediatrics.* (19th ed.) (pp. lxvii, p. 2610). Philadelphia, PA: Elsevier/Saunders.

Gast, G. C., Samsioe, G. N., Grobbee, D. E., Nilsson, P. M., & van der Schouw, Y. T. (2010). Vasomotor Symptoms, Estradiol Levels and Cardiovascular Risk Profile in Women. *Maturitas, 66*(3), 285–290. doi:10.1016/j.maturitas.2010.03.015.

Gil, M., Oliva, B., Timoner, J., Maciá, M. A., Bryant, V., & de Abajo, F. J. (2011). Risk of Meningioma Among Users of High Doses of Cyproterone Acetate as Compared with the General Population: Evidence from a Population-Based Cohort Study. *British Journal of Clinical Pharmacology, 72*(6), 965–968. doi:10.1111/j.1365-2125.2011.04031.x.

Giltay, E. J., & Gooren, L. J. (2000). Effects of Sex Steroid Deprivation/Administration On Hair Growth and Skin Sebum Production in Transsexual Males and Females. *The Journal of Clinical Endocrinology and Metabolism, 85*(8), 2913–2921.

Gooren, L., & Morgentaler, A. (2013). Prostate Cancer Incidence in Orchidectomised Male-To-Female Transsexual Persons Treated with Oestrogens. *Andrologia*. doi:10.1111/and.12208.

Gooren, L. J. (2014). Management of Female-To-Male Transgender Persons: Medical and Surgical Management, Life Expectancy. *Current Opinion in Endocrinology, Diabetes, and Obesity, 21*(3), 233–238. doi:10.1097/MED.0000000000000064.

Gooren, L. J., van Trotsenburg, M. A., Giltay, E. J., & van Diest, P. J. (2013). Breast Cancer Development in Transsexual Subjects Receiving Cross-Sex Hormone Treatment. *The Journal of Sexual Medicine, 10*(12), 3129–3134. doi:10.1111/jsm.12319.

Grynberg, M., Fanchin, R., Dubost, G., Colau, J. C., Brémont-Weil, C., Frydman, R., et al. (2010). Histology of Genital Tract and Breast Tissue After Long-Term Testosterone Administration in a Female-To-Male Transsexual Population. *Reproductive Biomedicine Online, 20*(4), 553–558. doi:10.1016/j.rbmo.2009.12.021.

Gulmez, S. E., Lassen, A. T., Aalykke, C., Dall, M., Andries, A., Andersen, B. S., et al. (2008). Spironolactone Use and the Risk of Upper Gastrointestinal Bleeding: A Population-Based Case-Control Study. *British Journal of Clinical Pharmacology, 66*(2), 294–299. doi:10.1111/j.1365-2125.2008.03205.x.

Hale, G. E., & Shufelt, C. L. (2015). Hormone Therapy in Menopause: An Update on Cardiovascular Disease Considerations. *Trends in Cardiovascular Medicine, 25*(6), 540–549. doi:10.1016/j.tcm.2015.01.008.

Hembree, W. C., Cohen-Kettenis, P., Delemarre-van de Waal, H. A., Gooren, L. J., Meyer, W. J., Spack, N. P., et al. (2009). Endocrine Treatment of Transsexual Persons: An Endocrine Society Clinical Practice Guideline.

The Journal of Clinical Endocrinology and Metabolism, 94(9), 3132–3154. doi:10.1210/jc.2009-0345.

Hiort, O. (2002). Androgens and Puberty. *Best Practice & Research. Clinical Endocrinology & Metabolism, 16*(1), 31–41. doi:10.1053/beem.2002.0178.

Hutchison, J. B. (1997). Gender-Specific Steroid Metabolism in Neural Differentiation. *Cellular and Molecular Neurobiology, 17*(6), 603–626.

Inki, P. (2007). Long-Term Use of the Levonorgestrel-Releasing Intrauterine System. *Contraception, 75*(Suppl. 6), S161–S166. doi:10.1016/j.contraception.2006.12.016.

Jacobstein, R., & Polis, C. B. (2014). Progestin-Only Contraception: Injectables and Implants. *Best Practice & Research. Clinical Obstetrics & Gynaecology, 28*(6), 795–806. doi:10.1016/j.bpobgyn.2014.05.003.

Jeppsson, S., Johansson, E. D., Ljungberg, O., & Sjöberg, N. O. (1977). Endometrial Histology and Circulating Levels Of Medroxyprogesterone Acetate (MPA), Estradiol, FSH and LH in Women with MPA Induced Amenorrhoea Compared with Women with Secondary Amenorrhoea. *Acta Obstetricia et Gynecologica Scandinavica, 56*(1), 43–48.

Kannel, W. B. (2002). The Framingham Study: Historical Insight on the Impact of Cardiovascular Risk Factors in Men Versus Women. *The Journal of Gender-Specific Medicine, 5*(2), 27–37.

Khera, M. (2013). Patients with Testosterone Deficit Syndrome and Depression. *Archivos Españoles de Urología, 66*(7), 729–736.

Kwiecien, M., Edelman, A., Nichols, M. D., & Jensen, J. T. (2003). Bleeding Patterns and Patient Acceptability of Standard or Continuous Dosing Regimens of a Low-dose Oral Contraceptive: A Randomized Trial. *Contraception, 67*(1), 9–13.

Lapauw, B., Taes, Y., Simoens, S., Van Caenegem, E., Weyers, S., Goemaere, S., et al. (2008). Body Composition, Volumetric and Areal Bone Parameters in Male-To-Female Transsexual Persons. *Bone, 43*(6), 1016–1021. doi:10.1016/j.bone.2008.09.001.

Laufer, L. R., Erlik, Y., Meldrum, D. R., & Judd, H. L. (1982). Effect of Clonidine on Hot Flashes in Postmenopausal Women. *Obstetrics and Gynecology, 60*(5), 583–586.

Lee, L. V., & Foody, J. M. (2008). Cardiovascular Disease in Women. *Current Atherosclerosis Reports, 10*(4), 295–302.

Light, A. D., Obedin-Maliver, J., Sevelius, J. M., & Kerns, J. L. (2014). Transgender Men Who Experienced Pregnancy After Female-To-Male Gender Transitioning. *Obstetrics and Gynecology, 124*(6), 1120–1127. doi:10.1097/AOG.0000000000000540.

Lips, P., van Kesteren, P. J., Asscheman, H., & Gooren, L. J. (1996). The Effect of Androgen Treatment on Bone Metabolism in Female-To-Male Transsexuals. *Journal of Bone and Mineral Research, 11*(11), 1769–1773. doi:10.1002/jbmr.5650111121.

Loibl, S., Schwedler, K., von Minckwitz, G., Strohmeier, R., Mehta, K. M., & Kaufmann, M. (2007). Venlafaxine is Superior to Clonidine as Treatment of Hot Flashes in Breast Cancer Patients—A Double-Blind, Randomized Study. *Annals of Oncology, 18*(4), 689–693. doi:10.1093/annonc/mdl478.

Marshall, W. A., & Tanner, J. M. (1969). Variations in Pattern of Pubertal Changes in Girls. *Archives of Disease in Childhood, 44*(235), 291–303.

Marshall, W. A., & Tanner, J. M. (1970). Variations in the Pattern of Pubertal Changes in Boys. *Archives of Disease in Childhood, 45*(239), 13–23.

Marshall, W. A., & Tanner, J. M. (1986). Puberty. In F. Falkner & J. M. Tanner (Eds.), *Human Growth: A Comprehensive Treatise* (2nd ed., pp. 171–209). New York: Plenum Press.

Matsui, S., Yasui, T., Tani, A., Kato, T., Uemura, H., Kuwahara, A., et al. (2014). Effect of Ultra-Low-Dose Estradiol and Dydrogesterone on Arterial Stiffness in Postmenopausal Women. *Climacteric, 17*(2), 191–196. doi:10.3109/13697137.2013.856399.

McGreevy, C., & Williams, D. (2011). Safety of Drugs Used in the Treatment of Osteoporosis. *Therapeutic Advances in Drug Safety, 2*(4), 159–172. doi:10.1177/2042098611411012.

Melmed, S., & Williams, R. H. (2011). *Williams Textbook of Endocrinology* (12th ed.). Philadelphia, PA: Elsevier/Saunders.

Meyer, W. J., Finkelstein, J. W., Stuart, C. A., Webb, A., Smith, E. R., Payer, A. F., et al. (1981). Physical and Hormonal Evaluation of Transsexual Patients During Hormonal Therapy. *Archives of Sexual Behavior, 10*(4), 347–356.

Meyer, W. J., Webb, A., Stuart, C. A., Finkelstein, J. W., Lawrence, B., & Walker, P. A. (1986). Physical and Hormonal Evaluation of Transsexual Patients: A Longitudinal Study. *Archives of Sexual Behavior, 15*(2), 121–138.

Morgan, M. L., Cook, I. A., Rapkin, A. J., & Leuchter, A. F. (2005). Estrogen Augmentation of Antidepressants in Perimenopausal Depression: A Pilot Study. *The Journal of Clinical Psychiatry, 66*(6), 774–780.

Mueller, A., & Gooren, L. (2008). Hormone-Related Tumors in Transsexuals Receiving Treatment with Cross-Sex Hormones. *European Journal of Endocrinology, 159*(3), 197–202. doi:10.1530/EJE-08-0289.

Mueller, A., Haeberle, L., Zollver, H., Claassen, T., Kronawitter, D., Oppelt, P. G., et al. (2010). Effects of Intramuscular Testosterone Undecanoate on Body Composition and Bone Mineral Density in Female-

To-Male Transsexuals. *The Journal of Sexual Medicine, 7*(9), 3190–3198. doi:10.1111/j.1743-6109.2010.01912.x.

Mueller, S. C., Grissom, E. M., & Dohanich, G. P. (2014). Assessing Gonadal Hormone Contributions to Affective Psychopathologies Across Humans and Animal Models. *Psychoneuroendocrinology, 46*, 114–128. doi:10.1016/j.psyneuen.2014.04.015.

Neumann, F., & Kalmus, J. (1991). Cyproterone Acetate in the Treatment of Sexual Disorders: Pharmacological Base and Clinical Experience. *Experimental and Clinical Endocrinology, 98*(2), 71–80. doi:10.105 5/s-0029-1211103.

Nieschlag, E., & Behre, H. M. (2004). *Testosterone: Action, Deficiency, Substitution* (3rd ed.). Cambridge, UK: Cambridge University Press.

Onalan, G., Onalan, R., Selam, B., Akar, M., Gunenc, Z., & Topcuoglu, A. (2005). Mood Scores in Relation to Hormone Replacement Therapies During Menopause: A Prospective Randomized Trial. *The Tohoku Journal of Experimental Medicine, 207*(3), 223–231.

Reyes, F. I., Boroditsky, R. S., Winter, J. S., & Faiman, C. (1974). Studies on Human Sexual Development. II. Fetal and Maternal Serum Gonadotropin and Sex Steroid Concentrations. *The Journal of Clinical Endocrinology and Metabolism, 38*(4), 612–617. doi:10.1210/jcem-38-4-612.

Rhees, R. W., Kirk, B. A., Sephton, S., & Lephart, E. D. (1997). Effects of Prenatal Testosterone on Sexual Behavior, Reproductive Morphology and LH Secretion in the Female Rat. *Developmental Neuroscience, 19*(5), 430–437.

Richards, C., & Seal, L. (2014). Trans People's Reproductive Options and Outcomes. *The Journal of Family Planning and Reproductive Health Care.* doi:10.1136/jfprhc-2013-100669.

Rossouw, J. E., Anderson, G. L., Prentice, R. L., LaCroix, A. Z., Kooperberg, C., Stefanick, M. L., et al. (2002). Risks and Benefits of Estrogen Plus Progestin in Healthy Postmenopausal Women: Principal Results from the Women's Health Initiative Randomized Controlled Trial. *JAMA, 288*(3), 321-333.

Rossouw, J. E., Prentice, R. L., Manson, J. E., Wu, L., Barad, D., Barnabei, V. M., .et al. (2007). Postmenopausal Hormone Therapy and Risk of Cardiovascular Disease by Age and Years Since Menopause. *JAMA, 297*(13), 1465-1477. doi: 10.1001/jama.297.13.1465

Ruetsche, A. G., Kneubuehl, R., Birkhaeuser, M. H., & Lippuner, K. (2005). Cortical and Trabecular Bone Mineral Density in Transsexuals After Long-Term Cross-Sex Hormonal Treatment: A Cross-Sectional Study. *Osteoporosis International, 16*(7), 791–798.

Saarikoski, S., Yliskoski, M., & Penttilä, I. (1990). Sequential Use of Norethisterone and Natural Progesterone in Pre-menopausal Bleeding Disorders. *Maturitas, 12*(2), 89–97.

Salpeter, S. R., Walsh, J. M., Greyber, E., & Salpeter, E. E. (2006). Brief report: Coronary Heart Disease Events Associated with Hormone Therapy in Younger And Older Women. A Meta-Analysis. *Journal of General Internal Medicine, 21*(4), 363–366. doi:10.1111/j.1525-1497.2006.00389.x.

Sassarini, J., & Lumsden, M. A. (2015). Oestrogen Replacement in Postmenopausal Women. *Age and Ageing, 44*(4), 551–558. doi:10.1093/ageing/afv069.

Seal, L. J. (2007). The Hormonal Management of Adults with Gender Dysphoria. In J. Barrett (Ed.), *Transexual and Other Disorders of Gender Identity: A Practical Guide to Management* (pp. 157–185). London: Radcliffe.

Seal, L. J. (2009). Testosterone Replacement Therapy. *Medicine International, 37*(9), 445–449.

Seal, L. J. (2015). A Review of the Physical and Metabolic Effects of Cross-Sex Hormonal Therapy in the Treatment of Gender Dysphoria. *Annals of Clinical Biochemistry.* doi:10.1177/0004563215587763.

Seal, L. J., Franklin, S., Richards, C., Shishkareva, A., Sinclaire, C., & Barrett, J. (2012). Predictive Markers for Mammoplasty and a Comparison of Side Effect Profiles in Transwomen Taking Various Hormonal Regimens. *The Journal of Clinical Endocrinology and Metabolism, 97*(12), 4422–4428. doi:10.1210/jc.2012-2030.

Simon, L., Kozák, L. R., Simon, V., Czobor, P., Unoka, Z., Szabó, Á., et al. (2013). Regional Grey Matter Structure Differences Between Transsexuals and Healthy Controls—A Voxel Based Morphometry Study. *PLoS One, 8*(12), e83947. doi:10.1371/journal.pone.0083947.

Swaab, D. F., Hofman, M. A., Lucassen, P. J., Purba, J. S., Raadsheer, F. C., & Van de Nes, J. A. (1993). Functional Neuroanatomy and Neuropathology of the Human Hypothalamus. *Anatomy and Embryology (Berlin), 187*(4), 317–330.

Swerdloff, R. S., & Odell, W. D. (1975). Hormonal Mechanisms in the Onset of Puberty. *Postgraduate Medical Journal, 51*(594), 200–208.

Sánchez-Chapado, M., Olmedilla, G., Cabeza, M., Donat, E., & Ruiz, A. (2003). Prevalence of Prostate Cancer and Prostatic Intraepithelial Neoplasia in Caucasian Mediterranean Males: An Autopsy Study. *Prostate, 54*(3), 238–247. doi:10.1002/pros.10177.

Tapanainen, J., Kellokumpu-Lehtinen, P., Pelliniemi, L., & Huhtaniemi, I. (1981). Age-Related Changes in Endogenous Steroids of Human Fetal Testis During Early and Midpregnancy. *The Journal of Clinical Endocrinology and Metabolism, 52*(1), 98–102. doi:10.1210/jcem-52-1-98.

Tracz, M. J., Sideras, K., Boloña, E. R., Haddad, R. M., Kennedy, C. C., Uraga, M. V., et al. (2006). Testosterone Use in Men and Its Effects on Bone Health. A Systematic Review and Meta-Analysis of Randomized Placebo-Controlled Trials. *The Journal of Clinical Endocrinology and Metabolism, 91*(6), 2011–2016. doi:10.1210/jc.2006-0036.

Turo, R., Smolski, M., Esler, R., Kujawa, M. L., Bromage, S. J., Oakley, N., et al. (2014). Diethylstilboestrol for the Treatment of Prostate Cancer: Past, Present and Future. *Scandinavian Journal of Urology, 48*(1), 4–14. doi:10.3109/21681805.2013.861508.

Van Caenegem, E., Wierckx, K., Taes, Y., Dedecker, D., Van de Peer, F., Toye, K., et al. (2012). Bone Mass, Bone Geometry, and Body Composition in Female-To-Male Transsexual Persons After Long-Term Cross-Sex Hormonal Therapy. *The Journal of Clinical Endocrinology and Metabolism, 97*(7), 2503–2511. doi:10.1210/jc.2012-1187.

Van Goozen, S. H., Cohen-Kettenis, P. T., Gooren, L. J., Frijda, N. H., & Van de Poll, N. E. (1995). Gender Differences in Behaviour: Activating Effects of Cross-Sex Hormones. *Psychoneuroendocrinology, 20*(4), 343–363.

van Kesteren, P., Lips, P., Gooren, L. J., Asscheman, H., & Megens, J. (1998). Long-Term Follow-Up of Bone Mineral Density and Bone Metabolism in Transsexuals Treated with Cross-Sex Hormones. *Clinical Endocrinology, 48*(3), 347–354.

van Kesteren, P. J., Asscheman, H., Megens, J. A., & Gooren, L. J. (1997). Mortality and Morbidity in Transsexual Subjects Treated with Cross-Sex Hormones. *Clinical Endocrinology, 47*(3), 337–342.

Vanderschueren, D., Laurent, M. R., Claessens, F., Gielen, E., Lagerquist, M. K., Vandenput, L., et al. (2014). Sex Steroid Actions in Male Bone. *Endocrine Reviews, 35*(6), 906–960. doi:10.1210/er.2014-1024.

Wang, C., Swerdloff, R. S., Iranmanesh, A., Dobs, A., Snyder, P. J., Cunningham, G., et al. (2000). Transdermal Testosterone Gel Improves Sexual Function, Mood, Muscle Strength, and Body Composition Parameters in Hypogonadal Men. *The Journal of Clinical Endocrinology and Metabolism, 85*(8), 2839–2853.

Watts, N. B., Notelovitz, M., Timmons, M. C., Addison, W. A., Wiita, B., & Downey, L. J. (1995). Comparison of Oral Estrogens and Estrogens Plus Androgen on Bone Mineral Density, Menopausal Symptoms, and Lipid-

Lipoprotein Profiles in Surgical Menopause. *Obstetrics and Gynecology, 85*(4), 529–537.

Wells, G., Tugwell, P., Shea, B., Guyatt, G., Peterson, J., Zytaruk, N., et al. (2002). Meta-Analyses of Therapies for Postmenopausal Osteoporosis. V. Meta-Analysis of the Efficacy of Hormone Replacement Therapy in Treating and Preventing Osteoporosis in Postmenopausal Women. *Endocrine Reviews, 23*(4), 529–539. doi:10.1210/er.2001-5002.

Willemse, P. H., Dikkeschei, L. D., Mulder, N. H., van der Ploeg, E., Sleijfer, D. T., & de Vries, E. G. (1988). Clinical and Endocrine Effects of Cyproterone Acetate in Postmenopausal Patients with Advanced Breast Cancer. *European Journal of Cancer & Clinical Oncology, 24*(3), 417–421.

Winter, J. S., & Faiman, C. (1972). Pituitary-Gonadal Relations in Male Children and Adolescents. *Pediatric Research, 6*(2), 126–135. doi:10.1203/00006450-197202000-00006.

World Health Organization Task Force on Methods for the Regulation of Male Fertility. (1990). Contraceptive Efficacy of Testosterone-Induced Azoospermia in Normal Men. *Lancet, 336*(8721), 955–959.

Woods, N. F., & Mitchell, E. S. (2005). Symptoms During the Perimenopause: Prevalence, Severity, Trajectory, and Significance in Women's Lives. *The American Journal of Medicine, 118*(Suppl. 12B), 14–24. doi:10.1016/j.amjmed.2005.09.031.

Zhou, J. N., Hofman, M. A., Gooren, L. J., & Swaab, D. F. (1995). A Sex Difference in the Human Brain and Its Relation to Transsexuality. *Nature, 378*(6552), 68–70. doi:10.1038/378068a0.

Zitzmann, M., Faber, S., & Nieschlag, E. (2006). Association of Specific Symptoms and Metabolic Risks with Serum Testosterone in Older Men. *The Journal of Clinical Endocrinology & Metabolism, 91*(11), 4335–4343. doi:10.1210/jc.2006-0401.

Further Reading

Barrett, J. D. (2007). *Transsexual and Other Disorders of Gender Identity: A Practical Guide to Management.* Abingdon, UK: Radcliffe.

Hembree, W. C., Cohen-Kettenis, P., Delemarre-van de Waal, H. A., Gooren, L. J., Meyer, W. J., Spack, N. P., et al. (2009). Endocrine Treatment of Transsexual Persons: An Endocrine Society Clinical Practice Guideline. *The Journal of Clinical Endocrinology & Metabolism, 94*(9), 3132–3154. doi:10.1210/jc.2009-0345.

Melmed, S., & Williams, R. H. (2011). *Williams Textbook of Endocrinology* (12th ed.). Philadelphia, PA: Elsevier/Saunders.

Seal, L. J. (2015). A Review of the Physical and Metabolic Effects of Cross-Sex Hormonal Therapy in the Treatment of Gender Dysphoria. *Annals of Clinical Biochemistry*. doi:10.1177/0004563215587763.

Wylie, K., Barrett, J., Besser, M., Bouman, W., Brain, C., Bridgman, M., et al. (2013). *Good Practice Guidelines for the Assessment and Treatment of Adults with Gender Dysphoria*. Retrieved from http://www.rcpsych.ac.uk/files/pdf-version/CR181.pdf

11

Chest Surgeries

Andrew Yelland

Introduction

The presence or absence of breast tissue is one of the physical second-ary sexual characteristics that identify a person as male or female. In Western society, the breast occupies a psychosocial position far greater than its physical size. As such, those seeking to reassign their gender often seek breast/chest surgery to help accomplish their aims. By alter-ing the volume of breast tissue present in any given individual, however, we must be cognisant of the fact that we alter the delicate balance of breast/chest wall anatomy; and that there are also psychological implica-tions to this.

Non-binary individuals who seek breast/chest surgery are looking for specific results to enable them to make their body as congruous as pos-sible with their experienced gender, and indeed the view any individual

A. Yelland (✉)
Nuffield Hospital Brighton, Brighton, UK

© The Author(s) 2017
C. Richards et al. (eds.), *Genderqueer and Non-Binary Genders*, Critical and Applied
Approaches in Sexuality, Gender and Identity, DOI 10.1057/978-1-137-51053-2_11

may take of their breast/chest may vary naturally during life. Relatively little has been published on breast surgery for bodies commonly gendered as male or female within a non-binary context, and so the author gives his opinion based upon clinical experience with a relatively limited number of patients who identify as non-binary seeking this surgery, although the number of non-binary patients is increasing.

Anatomy and Physiology

Most breast surgeons will acknowledge that a sound grounding in the anatomy and physiology of the breast is an essential pre-requisite for the safe and appropriate surgical intervention on the breast. It is important to have an understanding of not only the breast itself but the underlying structures such as muscle and fascia as well (see Fig. 11.1).

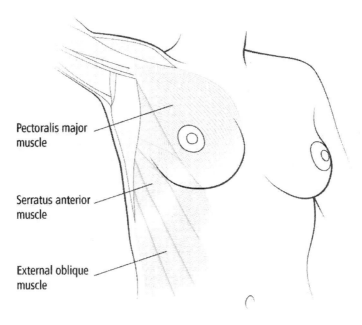

Fig. 11.1 Muscle and fascia in the breast region

Embryology

The breast develops as a differentiation of the cutaneous epithelium in the 6th to 8th weeks of pregnancy. This extends along the milk line extending from the axilla to groin. The breast tissue develops in the pectoral region primarily at the level of the fourth intercostal space, but supernumerary breast tissue can develop anywhere along this line from axilla to groin, although most frequently occurring just below the level of the inframammary crease.

Development

Prior to puberty, the nipple is located at the fourth intercostal space, and when the breast tissue first develops, it does so immediately beneath the nipple-areolar complex as a small disc. The birth-assigned female breast tissue will begin to develop between the ages of 9 and 14 and at this point develops into a conical structure, that is, with projection. This growth tends to be symmetrical, but does not need to be so, and developmental abnormalities can occur at this time resulting in unilateral hyperplasia or aplasia and more extensive abnormalities such as Poland syndrome. Breast hypertrophy can also occur during this period.

The development of the breast is classified into developmental stages by Tanner (Marshall & Tanner, 1969) (see Fig. 11.2).

Skin

As a skin appendage, clearly the breast is closely related to the skin, and the quality and elasticity of the skin can affect breast appearance. Striae, which are thinning of the epidermis, are found in patients post-pregnancy, or who have lost a significant amount of weight. This results in loss of skin elasticity, and this needs to be taken into consideration, for example, if the breast skin were expected to support the weight of an implant or even if the skin was resected during a mastopexy. In these situations, the skin may stretch resulting in a less aesthetically acceptable result in

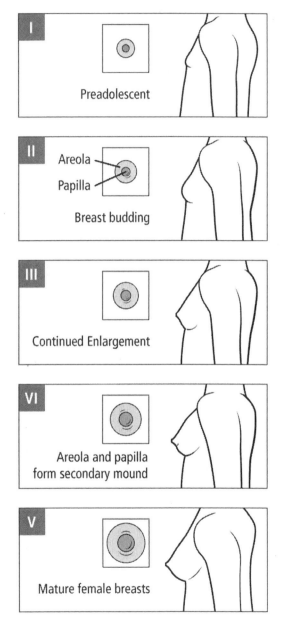

Fig. 11.2 The Tanner Stages

the case of the implant or re-ptosis in the case of mastopexy. The blood supply to the skin originates primarily from the sub-dermal plexus with communications to deeper lying perforator arteries running through the breast tissue. The sensation of the skin is segmental and derives from the dermatomes involved in breast development.

Breast Content

The content of breast tissue itself consists of two components; that of the actual milk-producing glandular secretory component called parenchyma; and fat. The fat content within a breast varies and is responsible for most of the bulk and soft consistency of the breast parenchyma. The actual glandular tissue consists of approximately 20 lobules which are radially arranged and which drain via a lactiferous duct to the nipple. The breast lactiferous ducts and lobules normally contain bacteria, most commonly Staphylococcus epidermidis which of course can play a role both in breast infection in conditions such as periductal mastitis and can be cultured from the capsule surrounding breast implants. For this reason, it is important to consider the use of antibiotics in breast surgery.

Blood Supply

The breast receives the blood predominantly from perforating branches of the internal mammary artery and from branches of the lateral thoracic artery entering via the axillary tail (see Fig. 11.3).

Fascia

The breast is contained within lines of the superficial fascia and lies on the deep fascia, which essentially separates the posterior aspect of the breast from the underlying pectoralis major muscle. The superficial fascia is essentially split, part of it lying immediately underneath the skin and a very thin layer lying on the immediate posterior surface of the breast. This latter layer abuts the deep fascia overlying the pectoralis major

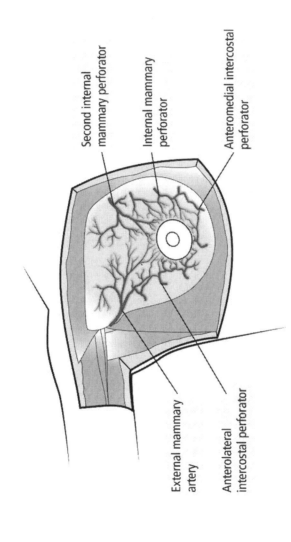

Second internal mammary perforator

Internal mammary perforator

Anteromedial intercostal perforator

External mammary artery

Anterolateral intercostal perforator

Fig. 11.3 Blood supply of the breast

muscle. Running through the breast are condensations of fascia known as Cooper's ligaments, which run from the deep fascia to the dermis, attaching the dermis to the overlying skin. The ligaments also reach into the deep fascia overlying the muscle. As these are not taut, they allow for movement in the breast, but with a loss of elasticity in the connective tissues, this can contribute to ptosis.

Underlying Musculature

The muscles underlying the breast consist of the pectoralis major muscle, the pectoralis minor muscle, and serratus anterior and external oblique with the pectoralis major underlying (see Fig. 11.1 above). The pectoralis major muscle has a wide sterno-clavicular origin, which can be divided into two components. The clavicular head arises from the medial half of the clavicle and runs almost horizontally. The sterno-costal head arises from the lateral part of the anterior surface of the manubrium, and body of the sternum on the deep surface of the muscle slips arises from the upper sixth costal cartilages. The muscle has a tendinous insertion into the neck of the humerus. The pectoralis minor has a bony origin on the third, fourth, and fifth ribs, and the muscle converges on the coracoid process of the scapula. The base of the breast is fairly constant extending from the second to the sixth ribs in the mid-clavicular line largely overlying the pectoralis major muscle and extending beyond that to the border to lie on the serratus anterior and external oblique muscles.

Nerve Supply of the Nipple-Areolar Complex

The nerve supply to the nipple-areolar complex is primarily from the fourth anterolateral intercostal nerve, but it is also served by the third and fifth intercostal nerves. There is also a contribution from the third, fourth, and fifth anterior medial intercostal nerves (see Fig. 11.4). This overlapping distribution explains why nipple sensation can be preserved in a number of surgical procedures. However, nipple-areolar sensation should always be mentioned to patients undergoing breast surgery as sensation appears to vary widely between individuals and to some degree to have a subjective variation.

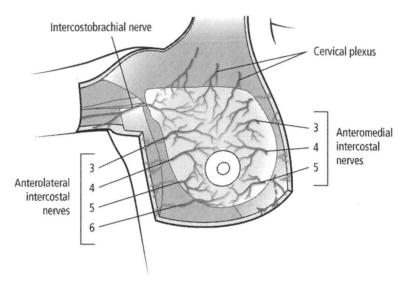

Fig. 11.4 Nerve supply to the breast

Preliminary Impression

Forming an impression about a patient begins with receipt of the referring letter from a clinician from the Gender Identity Clinic service (GICs). This may highlight certain characteristics, behaviour patterns, or specific desires the patient has already expressed. Often patients will also make contact by either telephone or email prior to consultation, and again this can be helpful in forming an opinion. The initial consultation is the first face-to-face meeting with the patient, and it is important that a good doctor-patient relationship is formed at this stage. Certainly, it is important that the patient realises that I have a genuine desire to help and will listen to specific thoughts and requests for the post-operative appearance. It is important for me to remember that surgery often represents a goal at the end of a process which may have started many years, or sometimes decades before. Often patients will attend with significant others or family for support which is necessary during the post-operative period at home in order to reduce the risk of complications and therefore optimise a good surgical outcome.

Body Mass Index

A number of institutions have introduced body mass index (BMI) limits under certain circumstances such as day case surgery. However, clinicians should be aware that weight gain can be used as a method to disguise gender and as such should be sensitive to the preoperative BMI of patients. It must be noted, however, that risks of surgery do increase with increasing BMI. There have been reported increases in the risk of deep vein thrombosis (DVT) and pulmonary embolism, infection rates (wound, urinary tract, and chest), and cardiac rhythm abnormalities in addition to the increased practical difficulties such as siting intravenous cannulae. It must also be noted that for vaginoplasty surgery the BMI needs to be within normal limits as the risk of neo-vaginal prolapse increases with increasing BMI. Similarly, there are BMI requirements for phalloplasty and metoidioplasty due to the possible complications associated with a high BMI. Specifically with regard to the result of chest reconstructive surgery, if patients intend to lose weight post-operatively as they are more comfortable with their gendered appearance, then the results may not be maintained by way of general loss of subcutaneous fat and to some degree breast parenchyma. It is also important to recognise that the larger a patient is, the more difficult it is to obtain the best results. Therefore, weight must be stable in the perioperative period.

Cross-Sex Hormone Treatment

Cross-sex hormone therapy has been reported to increase risk of blood clots in all patient groups. In patients undergoing genital reassignment surgery, it is common practice to stop hormone therapy 6 weeks preoperatively. This must be put into context with the fact that these patients are required to remain relatively immobile for a number of days post-operatively. Patients undergoing chest reconstructive surgery or augmentation mammoplasty, however, are able to be mobile immediately post-surgery and should therefore be encouraged to be so. It is not advised that surgeons stop cross-sex hormone therapy preoperatively (indeed this could also be difficult to time, given that depot injections are often used). Instead routine measures such as prophylaxis including compression stockings and hydration are advised. Reassuringly, to date the DVT rate has been very low.

Family History of Breast Cancer

A family history of breast cancer or related cancers has been an established part of breast surgical history taking for many years. Recent medical advances in this area have raised its profile further. Certainly a note should be made of such a family history. The risk of breast cancer developing in a transgender patient is reported not to be increased, but the scientific basis for this is limited (Brown & Jones, 2015). It is therefore advised that, as well as taking a family history and advising accordingly, a mammogram in all patients over 40 years of age should be undertaken. Some patients will have already undergone mammography as part of the National Health Service (NHS) breast cancer-screening programme in the United Kingdom, and this result may be accepted for a period of 12 months following its performance. Those patients with a proven genetic predisposition to develop breast cancer should have already been counselled with regard to their lifetime risk. It should be noted that natal males may also develop breast cancer, albeit at a lower rate than their female counterparts; and some breast cancers are associated with specific genetic changes.

Trans men and those non-binary people who were assigned female at birth will retain some breast tissue post-operatively and must be aware of the later potential risk for the development of breast cancer, however small. It is also useful to send all breast tissue for histological analysis in patients over the age of 40 as well as younger people with a previous history of breast problems or any other type of pertinent family history. To date, however, I have not detected any histological changes of relevance.

Trans women and those non-binary people who were assigned male at birth do have a lower breast cancer risk than their [female] birth-assigned counterparts—presumably due to the smaller amount of breast tissue present. In this context, the use of oestrogens does also increase the level of breast cancer risk, but again there is no significant data. Trans females will of course be invited to attend the National Health Service Breast Screening Programme and receive regular mammography from approximately the age of 50 to 70 (Public Health England, 2016); however, nonbinary people not registered with the NHS may not receive notification of this and may need to make individual arrangements via their general practitioner or family physician.

Clinical Examination

As part of the initial consultation, all patients will undergo a clinical examination. The aim of this is to assess the following elements in order to enable a discussion and selection of the most suitable surgical procedure.

Breast size and symmetry should be noted; symmetry needs particular care as the weight of tissue removed will therefore be different from each side. The presence of breast ptosis, the skin quality, and the nipple-areolar position will help to determine the suitability of the techniques that will be used. Body piercings or tattoos, which lie in the surgical field, should also be identified and discussed with the patient. In the author's experience, nipple piercing does not increase the risk of graft failure for the nipple-areola complex, but the patient should be made aware that this is a potential risk. It is always worth enquiring as to the patients' expectation and aims and any results they may have seen in others that they would like; or that they wish to avoid.

Operative Options

Breast Reduction

Breast reduction is a procedure with high patient satisfaction. This is because it leads to the resolution of both aesthetic and functional difficulties for patients with large breasts.

In the birth-assigned female population, it is important to ascertain the degree of reduction required. Often patients do request a significant reduction in size and it is important to discuss with them the degree to which they wish their breasts to be reduced. In this scenario, careful consideration must be given to the final shape and volume of the breast as the final result must accord with their self-perception and therefore ability to adjust to their new self-image.

It has been my experience, however, that a significant proportion of patients presenting for mastectomy and chest reconstructive surgery have undergone a breast reduction procedure earlier in their lives and have quite clearly wished for their breasts to be significantly smaller even at that point in time. For this reason, this section is included and it is important for the surgeon to understand the degree to which the patient would wish for their breasts to be made smaller as this can include very major reductions to say an A or AA cup or even "virtually flat".

It is not within the scope of this chapter to describe every method for performing bilateral reduction. The essential principles are, however, a reduction of the skin envelope including areolar diameter as well as the breast parenchyma. This can be achieved by either utilisation of a pedicle or the free nipple graft technique.

Free Nipple Graft Technique

This, in the author's practice, is reserved for those cases in which the breast is extremely large and more than a kilogram of breast tissue must be removed from each side. The intended nipple-areolar elevation is also well in excess of 10 cm rendering a pedicle-based procedure liable to failure. In terms of revising this to chest reconstruction, there is little to be considered other than that the scars from the previous reduction, which will be of an inverted T or anchor type pattern, should aim to be excised. The technique is in many ways similar to that of the free nipple graft chest reconstructive surgery.

Pedicle Techniques

Pedicle techniques include the inferior pedicle and superomedial pedicle techniques. In the author's opinion, the inferior pedicle gives more room for flexibility in terms of nipple repositioning and volume reduction with sculpting of the remaining breast tissue. It would certainly be the author's preference to use this technique if a patient were to request a reduction mammoplasty as, as it were, a first step towards considering chest reconstruction for the above-mentioned reasons.

The superomedial technique is perhaps used more frequently at the present time and can be utilised with either a more traditional inverted T or anchor-shaped incision or a short vertical scar technique such as the Lejour, which can also be accompanied by simultaneous liposuction (although simultaneous liposuction has produced volume deficits in certain areas of the breast).

In terms of revision, the short vertical scar technique with its inferior pole volume loss and rouching of the skin is, in the author's opinion, more likely to present a difficulty with revision than the more traditional forms of reduction.

Mastectomy and Chest Reconstruction

For most patients, hormonal manipulation has relatively little effect on the volume of breast tissue. As an impression, the author feels that maximum effect of hormone therapy has been attained within a year of treatment. The quality of the breast tissue does appear to be altered in favour of less firm/dense tissue, which is then easier to manipulate. Of course non-binary individuals may not wish to consider hormone therapy. The absence of hormone therapy does not affect the final outcome, but the surgeon should be aware that the breast tissue may be firmer. Surgery therefore remains the primary mechanism to achieve a reduction in breast volume and/or masculine shape.

The aim of chest reconstructive surgery in this situation is to reduce the overall breast to attain a more masculine result. This is achieved by:

* Reducing breast volume
* Reducing skin envelope
* Obliterating the inframammary fold
* Obliterating the lateral impression of the breast
* Reducing areolar diameter
* Reducing nipple bud projection and diameter

* Repositioning the new nipple-areolar complex
* Ideally keeping scarring to a minimum
* Preserving sensation where possible

Skin elasticity must be borne in mind in these cases in particular; as there may have been many years of "binding", that is, compressing the breast tissue to disguise breast volume to the casual observer. Physically, the long-term compression of skin can lead to relatively poor blood supply and skin which is therefore at increased risk of wound breakdown and necrosis. Most cases fall short of this, but patients should be advised to stop binding prior to surgery to obviate this risk if damaged skin is noted.

In their seminal paper on gender confirming surgery, Monstrey et al. (2008) describe an algorithm of five different techniques (semicircular; transareolar; concentric circular; extended concentric; free nipple graft) to achieve a cosmetically acceptable chest. This is often referred to as the Ghent Algorithm. The techniques described are valid, but in only two, that is, the free nipple graft (double incision technique) and concentric circular (peri-areolar) are frequently used in my practice and result in reproducible cosmetically acceptable results. Liposuction alone may be used in very small-breasted individuals or as an adjunct to other surgical techniques. It is important, regardless of technique, to take care to preserve enough subcutaneous fat and glandular tissue to maintain a pleasing contour. Failure to do so leaves an unpleasant cosmetic result and a difficult situation to correct.

Having trained in general and plastic surgery, and having undertaken mastectomy in the circumstances of malignancy and gynaecomastia, the author believes it is important to recognise that surgery in a transgender healthcare setting is different and requires a different approach. The chest must be as aesthetically pleasing as is surgically possible to the non-binary person after surgery. In the cancer setting, I would tend to use an oblique incision to keep this away from the midline so that the theoretical opening up of other lymphatic channels does not occur and the scar is also kept away from the visible "decollotage" area. I also find that the in-setting of flap reconstructions tend to sit better in this direction. The axilla can also be easily approached via this incision. In gynaecomastia, the aim is very much minimal incision and so I tend to at least initially consider liposuction and if sufficient tissue remains to consider subcutaneous resection of the remaining tissue via a circumareolar incision. Subcutaneous mastectomy can be considered de novo using this technique. However, if there is sufficient tissue and also poor skin quality and/or the presence of significant ptosis, then I would tend to utilise the double incision technique.

Double Incision Technique

The author utilises this procedure for the majority of cases. The technique removes both skin and breast parenchyma and allows a good access to the plane overlying the fascia over the pectoralis major muscle. Certainly, to the author's eyes, breast volumes estimated to exceed 200 to 250 g should be treated utilising this method.

The procedure itself involves harvesting the nipple-areolar complex as a full-thickness skin graft. The breast is then amputated and the nipple area complex grafted into its new location of the chest wall. The author's preference is to place the lower part of the incision at the inframammary fold. If it is important to use clinical judgement, however, concerning repositioning of the nipple-areolar complex. No suction drains are used in this procedure as in the author's experience, the incidence of postoperative serum is minor and the discomfort and potential infection risk of drains outweigh the benefits.

Peri-areolar Technique

Contrastingly, I would estimate that I utilise the peri-areolar technique much less frequently, probably in no more than 5% to 7% of cases. The procedure involves a double concentric circular technique similar to that described by Davidson (1979). The nipple is preserved on a superior dermo-glandular pedicle and is resized. The remaining lower part of the incision enables resection of the parenchymal tissue, and it is important to note that there is probably less in the way of ability to reposition the nipple area complex utilising this technique. Some surgeons use an extended incision laterally from the concentric circular incision, but the author does not favour this particular procedure as it results in a visible scar which is in a relatively prominent position detracts from the overall aesthetic result.

Liposuction

Liposuction can be utilised either in the primary treatment of excess breast volume or in the refashioning of certain areas of breast tissue—for example, laterally towards the axilla.

The author's preference is to use the tumescent technique as described by Klein (1990). This involves the use of tumescence solution and micro-cannulas. In this case, the breast is approached via two stab incisions, one placed centrally beneath the inframammary fold and a second more laterally towards the anterior axillary line. The area is infiltrated with the tumescent solution and tissue aspirated using a suction pump. Post-operatively, the patient should wear a compression garment and expect the loss of the haemo-serous fluid for a period of 24–48 hours. While this is a viable technique, in the authors experience this should be relatively sparingly used as a primary technique. Cases suitable for primary lipo-suction alone would include those with a relatively small breast volume (less than 200 g); good position of the nipple-areolar complex; good skin elasticity; and a relatively fatty breast, that is, one in which there is not a significant proportion of dense fibrous glandular tissue. It may however be a useful adjunct to the more formal surgical procedures already men-tioned above.

Nipple-Areolar Procedures

It has already been noted that during the techniques of double incision and peri-areolar, the nipple-areola complexes are by definition resized. In the double incision technique, the nipple is removed and, as stated, the full thickness skin graft reduces the areolar diameter. The author's preference is not to alter the nipple bud itself as this often retracts, and provided the graft has been taken thin enough, it assumes a more masculine appearance. In the peri-areolar technique, again the areolar diameter is reduced. In the author's experience, it is often necessary to shorten the bud projection by amputation to obtain a more masculine appearance.

Revision, Causes for, and Complications

Inadequate or Excessive Resection

The aim of chest reconstructive surgery must be to create a smooth contour of tissue which resembles the male form. Either excessive or inadequate tissue excision will detract from this.

Seroma

A seroma is a pocket of clear serous fluid that sometimes develops in the body after surgery. When small blood vessels are ruptured, blood plasma can seep out; inflammation caused by dying injured cells also contributes to the fluid. The build-up of fluid in the subglandular space, or space between the tissue flap and pectoralis major muscle, is caused by the transudation of fluid across the area where the breast has either been disturbed (augmentation) or removed (chest reconstruction). Suction drainage has traditionally been used to treat this and most recently low-pressure systems. Traditionally, relatively high-pressure suction drains were used following surgical intervention. "Redivac" drains typically exerted pressures in the region of 100 mm mercury. In the 1980s, numerous papers demonstrated less in the way of post-operative seroma formation with low-pressure systems. Drains can be unpleasant to remove and are a potential portal for infection. I have never used drainage in primary augmentation and rapidly abandoned its use in mastectomy and chest reconstruction. After augmentation, I suggest a supportive sports bra; And after mastectomy and in chest reconstruction, in which moderate compression can be achieved by the use of lumbar support-type garment, I can only recall one case of troublesome seroma accumulation, and it was unclear whether drainage would have helped in this case, as there were other contributing factors. My impression is that seromatous accumulation is greatest in volume and more frequent in the peri-areolar version of chest reconstruction as opposed to the double incision approach.

Dog-Ears

Dog-ears are a pouting of the skin, usually found at the lateral end of the long incision in the double incision technique, although it can occur medially. They often appear more prominent from above than when viewed at a distance and can therefore be disconcerting for the patient. They can occur if the scar is insufficient in length or some parenchyma remains deep to the scar at this point. Most dog-ears will settle with time if minor, and gentle massage may be used without further intervention. But if this is not successful, then further excision of the underlying subcutaneous tissue will correct the prominence.

Revisional Surgery from Other Surgeons

The author has encountered a number of cases where revision has been required and almost exclusively this has resulted from the use of the peri-areolar or extended peri-areolar techniques, where perhaps the double incision technique would have been better applied. This has tended to result in uneven tissue resection—often too much centrally and too little laterally. In this situation, I have tended to utilise the double incision technique to correct the problem.

Ethnic Considerations

It should be noted that the scars of the double incision technique are relatively lengthy and to some degree prone to stretching and hypertrophy. In dark-skinned individuals, the author's preference is to use a subcuticular prolene suture. It is important to advise the patients at the outset that there may well be hypertrophic keloid formation and also patchy depigmentation of any grafted nipple-areola complex. These scar complications can be ameliorated to some degree using the normal methods; that is, non-absorbable suture use, timely suture removal, scar massage, and use of silicone-based scar treatments, as well as the longer-term wound support using micropore tape. If the above treatments are unsuccessful, then there may be the need for intradermal steroid injection or formal secondary excision and resuture.

Complications of Surgery

Infection

This appears to be relatively rare in all types of surgery. The author's infection rate is less than 0.5%. Antibiotics are used at induction of anaesthesia, and following surgery, a further two doses are administered.

Venous Thromboembolism

The occurrence of DVT appears very rare as patients are mobilised immediately post-operatively. Standard DVT prophylaxis includes the use of below-knee Thrombo Embolic Deterrent (TED) stockings, but I do not utilise low molecular weight heparin and do not encourage patients to stop their cross-sex hormone treatment prior to surgery.

Revision

In the author's experience, lateral "dog-ears" appear relatively infrequently. To date, the majority of revisions in the author's practice are those of shortening the nipple bud. This occurs with both the peri-areolar and double incision techniques. In the peri-areolar technique, if the nipple bud appears likely to remain too long, this can be shortened during the procedure by amputation. Following the double incision technique, the free nipple graft can remain large despite attempts to encourage its flattening. In such cases, the bud will require amputation as a secondary procedure in the outpatient department under local anaesthetic.

A central "dimple" can seem to appear in patients who had preoperatively a relatively narrow intermammary distance or symmastia or where the breast tissue weight resected was very large—that is, in excess of 1 kg per side. The author's preference to correct this central dimple is by excising any redundant skin bilaterally and extending the incisions across the midline, double-breasting the skin in this position by de-epithelialising the central bridge of skin and closing the peripheral incisions over this. This stops the shadowing of light at this position.

Long-Term Results

The techniques as mentioned above seem to have resulted in durable long-term results. The only exception concerns those patients who subsequently lose a significant amount of weight (more than one stone) or greater. These patients are advised that there is likely to be deterioration of the cosmetic result due to loss of weight affecting their overall body habitus.

References

Brown, G. R., & Jones, K. T. (2015). Incidence of Breast Cancer in a Cohort of 5,135 Transgender Veterans. *Breast Cancer Research and Treatment, 149*(1), 191–198.

Davidson, B. A. (1979). Concentric Circle Operation for Massive Gynaecomastia to Excise the Redundant Skin. *Plastic Reconstructive Surgery, 63*(3), 350–354.

Monstrey, S., Selvaggi, G., Ceulemans, P., Van Landuyt, K., Bowman, C., Blondeel, P., et al. (2008). Chest-Wall Contouring Surgery in Female-to-Male Transsexual: A New Algorithm. *Plastic Reconstructive Surgery, 121*(3), 849–859.

Klein, J. A. (1990). The Tumescent Technique. Anesthesia and Modified Liposuction Technique. *Dermatology Clinics, 8*(3), 425–437.

Marshall, W. A., & Tanner, J. M. (1969, June). Variations in Pattern of Pubertal Changes in Girls. *Archives of Diseases in Childhood, 44*(235), 291–303.

Public Health England. (2016). *NHS Breast Screening Programme* (4th ed.). NHSBSP Publication No. 49. London: DoH.

Further Reading

NHS Choices. (2017). *Breast Enlargement*. Retrieved February 22, 2017, from http://www.nhs.uk/Conditions/cosmetic-treatments-guide/Pages/breast-enlargement.aspx

Monstrey, S., Selvaggi, G., Ceulemans, P., Van Landuyt, K., Bowman, C., Blondeel, P., et al. (2008). Chest-Wall Contouring Surgery in Female-to-Male Transsexual: A New Algorithm. *Plastic Reconstructive Surgery*, *121*(3), 849–859.

Public Health England. (2016). *NHS Breast Screening Programme* (4th ed.). NHSBSP Publication No. 49. London: DoH.

12

Surgery for Bodies Commonly Gendered as Male

James Bellringer

Introduction

Historical Perspective

Surgery to achieve a neuter gender appears to have been practised back in ancient civilisations. Indeed, it is a matter of debate whether the brother of the god Osiris, Seth, was an eunuch (Pinch, 2004). There are also numerous references to eunuchs in the Bible and many other ancient texts, for example, the writings of Herodotus and Xenophon. The operations themselves were varied; the most drastic form was the removal of both testes and the penis, although excision of only the testes, or only the penis, is also described. Probably more frequently, especially in young pre-pubertal boys, the testes were crushed, or the spermatic cords ligated, from the outside, with the subsequent loss of the testes. These lesser procedures, whilst still to modern ears barbaric, had at least the advantage

J. Bellringer (✉)
Parkside Hospital, London, UK

© The Author(s) 2017
C. Richards et al. (eds.), *Genderqueer and Non-Binary Genders*, Critical and Applied
Approaches in Sexuality, Gender and Identity, DOI 10.1057/978-1-137-51053-2_12

that the mortality of the subjects was less than 80%. The majority of subjects did not come to castration voluntarily and were typically prisoners captured in wars or slaves. There is, however, some evidence that undergoing castration in ancient China, which in that society was the most radical form where all the external genitalia were removed with a single knife cut, in addition to being one of the Five Punishments, was also regarded as a way of gaining employment in the Imperial Court; so it might be that some individuals came forward without duress (Scheidel, 2009). As above, the operative mortality of complete excision of the external genitalia was around 80%, presumably from a combination of bleeding and sepsis, but in the longer term, most had difficulties with micturition, probably as a result of urethral stenosis. The use of a lead tube to maintain the patency of the urethra is described, and it may be assumed that other tubular devices were also employed, such as bamboo.

Although those who had been castrated in these times may not normally have chosen a neuter gender identity, there is no doubt that they occupied a separate role from men and women in society, sometimes attaining high status. For example, in the Byzantine court, certain posts were available only to eunuchs, including that of chamberlain to the emperor. From the point of view of sexual function, eunuchs also appear to have had a separate role from both men and women, as evidenced by the description of Alexander the Great's relationship with [the eunuch] Bagoas, which is described separately from his numerous hetero- and homosexual encounters. Furthermore, those assigned to guard harems may well have been sexually active with the women they were meant to be protecting, as one story from the Arabian Nights relates. Certainly, some who had undergone crushing of the testes might have retained sufficient testicular tissue for hormone production sufficient to support erectile function, although they would have been sterile.

In medieval Europe, bilateral orchidectomy was occasionally chosen by some, who felt that it would enable them to lead a more pious and pure life. It could certainly reasonably be argued that these individuals were undergoing castration voluntarily to lead a life different to either men or women, and thus might be regarded as people who had requested surgery to achieve a non-binary gender. The same is almost certainly not true of young boys who were submitted to orchidectomy to preserve their singing voices.

From a surgical point of view, the likeliest techniques for these orchidectomies would have been crushing of the testes from without ('emasculators' remain in regular veterinary use for castrating farm animals) or ligation of the spermatic cords also from outside by the application of a tight ligature around the neck of the scrotum. Open procedures, where the testes were removed by an incision in the scrotum with the spermatic cords ligated directly, almost certainly did take place. However, these would have carried a significantly higher morbidity from bleeding and infection, and would not have been performed as frequently, although there was significant variation geographically. These open procedures would be done by a direct incision in the scrotum to expose the testes, and then dissection to reveal the spermatic cords, which would be ligated. Removal of the entire external genitalia with a sharp instrument (as practised in ancient China) continues even today in modern India, where it is practised among the *Hijra*. The resulting open wound is packed with turmeric and other spices (to prevent bleeding and infection) and heals by granulation. There is a high incidence of urethral problems in this group, principally from urethral stenosis.

Modern Surgical Options

Genital surgery for people who do not identify as their birth-assigned sex has more recently been undertaken on trans women who have sought such surgeries to align their bodies with their internal sense of self as women (Bellringer, 2007). These groups of [trans] women may opt for a variety of procedures including orchidectomy; the removal of the penis and testicles without the creation of a vagina (called a cosmesis or cosmetic vulvoplasty); or the above and the creation of a vagina. Crucially, in all cases where the person's core identity is female, it is simply that her circumstances or wishes align with a certain type of surgery or body. For example, a person with limited mobility may opt not to have a vaginoplasty as the regular dilation of the neo-vagina with an acrylic stent necessitated by this surgery would be impractical. Naturally, this pragmatic consideration is not reflective of her core identity as a woman. Further, some trans women do not feel that they need to have a vagina simply because they are a woman. Just as her genetically produced penis is not constitutive of her as a woman; so, she argues, she is not constituted as a woman by a surgically produced vagina. Other trans women take a different view feeling that a vagina is a vital part of their female self.

These practical considerations also hold true for non-binary people; however, non-binary people may also wish to have genitalia, which is neither traditionally 'female' (i.e. a vagina with a labia) nor male (i.e. a penis and testicles) as this non-binary genitalia matches their non-binary identity. It is to the various surgical options available which we now turn.

Genital Surgery

'Standard' genital surgery for trans women can conveniently be subdivided into its component parts. These are *bilateral orchidectomy; vaginoplasty; penectomy; urethral meatoplasty; clitoroplasty; and labioplasty;* Other surgical options for non-binary people include *penile minimisation* and *testicular and scrotal ablation.* We shall consider these in turn:

The vast majority of trans women request the 'full' operation detailed above, although some ask for only some parts; typically bilateral orchidectomy (removal of both testes) only; or a 'cosmetic' procedure where no vaginoplasty (creation of a vagina) is performed but female external genitalia are created. In the author's experience, patients with a non-binary gender identity usually opt for either orchidectomy alone, or a 'cosmetic' procedure. Whilst technically feasible either by using a bowel segment to form the vaginal lining or by using scrotal skin left redundant after an orchidectomy, none so far has requested vaginoplasty with the preservation of the penis, although one trans man asked for vaginal widening after a phalloplasty (construction of a penis), so the desire to have both penis and vagina for sexual function can occur. A very small number of patients have requested penectomy and urethral meatoplasty with the preservation of the testes, which would then be moved up into the abdomen; this is technically feasible, but the author has so far dissuaded the patients from taking this option. This is because, although the testes would still produce normal testosterone levels, they would no longer be palpable, and there would be a risk of a subsequent testicular tumour remaining undetected until a very late stage. As the patients who have enquired about this option thus far also wanted testosterone ablation, they have been persuaded that a bilateral orchidectomy is a medically safer option.

Bilateral Orchidectomy

Where performed in isolation, this may usually be done through a scrotal incision. This is normally placed in the midline raphe, as the resulting scar is usually far less visible than a transverse incision. The Dartos muscle is divided over each testis (see Fig. 12.1), and the testis is delivered (see Fig. 12.2). Dissection should then continue along the spermatic cord on each side as far as the external inguinal ring, where the cord is divided. A single transfixion suture is adequate for haemostasis. The ligated spermatic cord remnant on each side should be allowed to retract into the inguinal canal, and this may require it to be gently freed from the surrounding soft tissue. The spermatic cord is particularly prone to the formation of painful neuromas, and if the ligated end is not within the inguinal canal, this may need to be removed subsequently. This also applies where the orchidectomy is performed as part of a more extensive procedure.

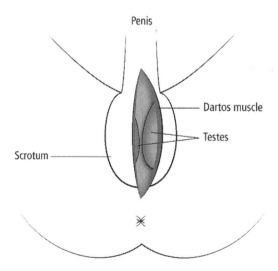

Fig. 12.1   Illustration of the position of Dartos muscle layer

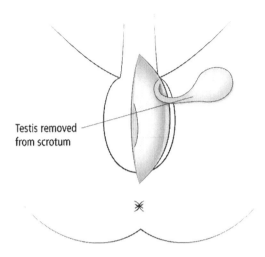

Fig. 12.2 Removal of the testis

After both testes are removed, the scrotum is closed in layers with absorbable sutures. The procedure may usually be performed on a day case basis. The commonest complication is a haematoma in the scrotum, which usually results from bleeding from the Dartos muscle layer.

Vaginoplasty

A vaginoplasty has two parts; first the creation of a cavity in the pelvis and then the lining of that cavity with an epithelium. In anatomical males, there is a potential space, the plane of Denonvilliers, between the rectum and the prostate, which may be entered through the perineum. Once this space is entered, it may be lengthened and widened without risk to the other pelvic organs. There are two techniques for entering the plane of Denonvilliers. First, the skin of the perineum is incised. The urethra lies subcutaneously in the perineum, surrounded by the bulbospongiosus muscle, and it is dissected free from the surrounding tissues. At this point, the commonest technique is to dissect the bulbospongiosus muscle away from the urethra until its origin in a fibrous attachment at the front of the perineal body is reached. This is incised transversely, allowing a fingertip to pass through onto the apex of the prostate gland. Either a finger or a blunt instrument is then placed in the rectum to act as a guide for the finger at the apex of the prostate, and the original finger at the apex of the prostate is then gently introduced blindly into the plane. Once past the point where the rectum and prostate cease to be in contact, metal retractors may be introduced, and the vaginal cavity deepened and widened.

By contrast, the author's preferred technique is to place a sound in the bladder, which is used to push the prostate down towards the operator. The apex of the prostate is identified by palpation, and sharp dissection under direct vision passes through the perineal body onto the prostate. Once the plane of Denonvilliers has been identified, metal retractors may be inserted as the bladder sound is removed, and these enter the space without damage to the rectum. The space can then be widened and deepened by blunt dissection.

Both techniques carry a risk of injury to the rectum, but this appears to be less in the second technique described presumably because the 'danger point' where the rectum and prostate are in close apposition is approached under direct vision. If damage does occur, the rectum may be repaired, but there is an incidence of subsequent recto-vaginal fistula, which typically is reported at between 0.5 and 1.5% (Lawrence, 2006).

Once the cavity is made, it needs to be lined with an epithelial tissue—in the vast majority of cases, this is skin, but bowel segments may also be used. In the majority of uncircumcised birth-assigned males, there is sufficient skin on the penis alone to line a vagina of 15 cm. In such patients, the intact skin tube may simply be inverted into the cavity after the end of the tube (originally the prepuce) has been closed. Where there is insufficient penile skin to line the vagina, it may be augmented by skin from elsewhere. The scrotum is the usual tissue donor in this regard, as it is directly in the area, and is usually redundant following an orchidectomy. The author's preference is to use a vascularised island flap based on the posterior scrotal vessels, but worldwide it is more usual to use a free graft. The advantage of the latter technique is that the fat is removed from the donor skin before it is used; and also the hair follicles. In the author's experience, intra-operative epilation is seldom complete, and pre-operative epilation by laser or electrolysis is to be preferred. The use of a vascularised island flap requires pre-operative depilation to avoid lifelong issues with continuing hair growth in the neo-vagina. Rarely, free skin grafts from abdomen and thigh may also be used.

Where there is, even using scrotal skin, insufficient skin for the vaginal lining, bowel segments may be employed. A segment of bowel is isolated on its vascular pedicle, one end is closed, and the other brought down to be anastomosed to the perineal skin. The commonest segment is the sigmoid colon, although segments of right colon and detubularised ileum may also be used. These operations require an abdominal approach, which nowadays will usually be performed laparoscopically in addition to the perineal and pelvic dissection; and the increased complexity leads to increased risk of complications. Even in the best hands, breakdown of the anastomosis between the two ends of bowel left after the "vaginal" segment is isolated occurs in the region of 1% of operations. In the longer term, many patients experience mucous discharge which can be troublesome, and there is a risk after 15 years of developing defunction enteritis; which is a condition where the bowel segment which is no longer in contact with the faecal stream becomes inflamed. In severe cases, the resulting pain and discharge have required removal of the bowel segment. For these reasons, it is the author's opinion that bowel segment vaginoplasty should be reserved for the very few cases where insufficient skin exists for skin tube vaginoplasty, or the skin tube fails. It is possible that this might apply in some non-binary individuals, although the author has not yet seen any such cases.

Clitoroplasty

A sensate clitoris may be fashioned from part of the glans penis, dissected away from the remainder of the penis on its own neurovascular bundle. The original technique described by Rubin (1993) where the glans penis was dissected out on a pedicle formed from the urethra has largely been replaced by the technique described by Fang, Chen, and Ma (1992). It relies on the fact that the nerves and blood vessels to the glans penis run separately from the vessels which supply the skin and erectile tissue of the penis in a layer between Buck's fascia and the tunica albuginea of the corpora (see Fig. 12.3). A piece of the glans can be dissected away from the end of the penis, and then dissected back to the pubis, with preservation of the nerve and blood supply. If care

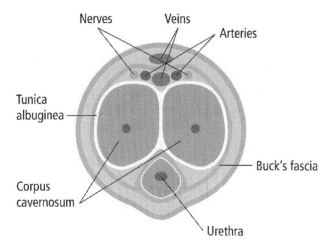

Fig. 12.3   Cross-section of the penis

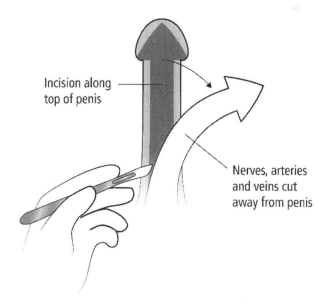

Fig. 12.4   Preservation of long pedicle

is taken to preserve the long pedicle (see Fig. 12.4), the piece of tissue from the glans can then be placed in a similar position to the birth-assigned female clitoris.

Labioplasty

Labioplasty is usually performed as part of either 'full' genital reconstruction, where a vagina is made, or as part of a cosmetic operation, where no vagina is made, but the genitalia are reconstructed to resemble cisgender female external genitalia. There are two components to the birth-assigned female labia; the labia majora, which are fleshy mounds on either side of the vagina and urethra, and the labia minora, which are relatively thin structures which form as a continuation of the clitoral prepuce and lie inside the two labia majora. From the point of view of construction, labia majora—when penectomy, orchidectomy, and urethral shortening are done—involve merely removing redundant scrotal tissue and closing the wounds to result in bilateral labia which resemble cisgender female labia reasonably closely (see Figs. 12.5, 12.6, and 12.7).

The labia minora are more difficult to construct. Probably, the commonest technique is to leave 1 cm of prepuce attached to the piece of glans penis used for a clitoroplasty, and then fold these down alongside the new urethral opening as a double layer of skin. This technique is practised particularly in Thailand (e.g. Watanayusaki, 2015). It produces cosmetically very satisfactory labia minora, but reduces the skin available for vaginoplasty, if that is to be done at the same time. In the author's practice, smaller skin folds are produced when the skin is brought down

Incision down
outer wall

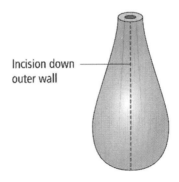

Fig. 12.5 Incision down outer wall

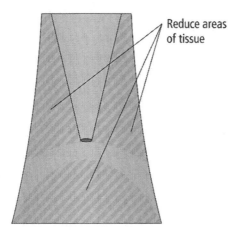

Reduce areas
of tissue

Fig. 12.6 Reduction of tissue areas

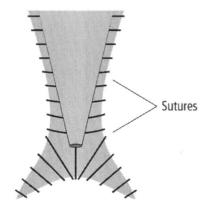

Sutures

Fig. 12.7 Sutures

alongside the new urethra, and these appear to be satisfactory for most patients.

Non-binary patients usually do not want their reconstructed genitalia to resemble either cisgender male or female genitalia, and therefore an attempt usually needs to be made to avoid creating labia minora (and certainly doing so from penile prepuce would not be indicated, unless the patient specified that that is what they wanted). Producing an entirely flat perineum with only a urethral meatus is all but impossible in most patients. First, the urethra needs to be divided in the area of the bulbar urethra, which typically lies 1–2 cm inside from the perineal skin, and second it is difficult to eliminate completely the appearance of labia majora, at least if the penis is also removed, although they can be minimised by the removal of much of the subcutaneous fat in this area.

Penile Minimisation

The author has had requests from non-binary patients to shorten the penis, but leave the remainder of the genitalia intact. This may be achieved relatively easily. A subcoronal incision is made on the penis (typically under tourniquet to minimise bleeding). The penis may then be degloved, by dissecting the skin tube back down to the root of the penis. Buck's fascia is then incised bilaterally and the neurovascular bundle is dissected away from the corpora cavernosa for the desired degree of shortening (see Figs. 12.8, 12.9, and 12.10). Ventrally, the urethra is dissected away from the corpora over the same length. A ring of tunica albuginea may then be excised from both corpora. The cut ends of the tunica are then joined with sutures, giving a shortening of the penis. If desired, the penis may also be narrowed along its shaft by excision of elliptical segments of tunica albuginea on each side.

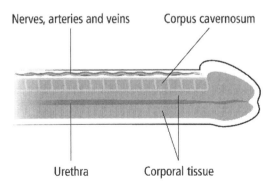

Fig. 12.8   Shortening process

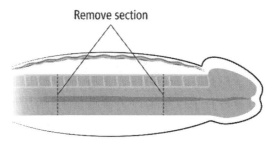

Fig. 12.9 Shortening process

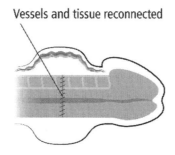

Fig. 12.10 Shortening process

Testicular and Scrotal Ablation

A very few patients request the removal of the testes and also scrotum, with retention of a normal penis. The author's experience of such cases is limited to two; one of whom achieved an orchidectomy by placing a tourniquet around the neck of the scrotum (which later required a formal orchidectomy in hospital); and one of whom had undergone an orchidectomy under local anaesthetic by a nurse working outside a hospital. In both cases, the patients requested excision of the scrotal skin, and in both, the spermatic cords bilaterally had formed painful neuromas which needed revision. After orchidectomy, excision of the residual scrotum is relatively simple. A lozenge-shaped area of skin is marked beginning ventrally on the penis, and extending to the perineal skin (see Fig. 12.11). The lateral margins of the 'lozenge' include the scrotum, which is dissected free from the remaining subcutaneous tissues and removed (see Fig. 12.12). In both cases, in the author's experience,

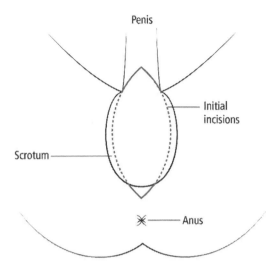

Fig. 12.11   Testicular and scrotal ablation

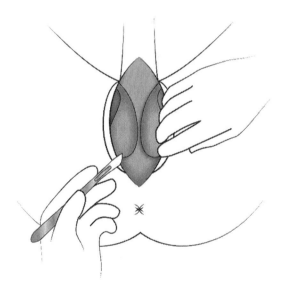

Fig. 12.12   Testicular and scrotal ablation

it was possible to identify the previously divided spermatic cords and dissect them back into the inguinal canal bilaterally, where they were re-ligated, but clearly, in a patient without a history of previous orchidectomy, both testes

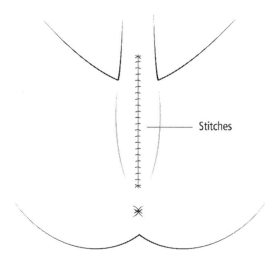

Fig. 12.13 Testicular and scrotal ablation

may be removed as described earlier. In the author's experience, it has been possible to close the resulting defect directly without excessive tension (see Fig. 12.13).

Referral for Surgery for Non-binary Individuals

Any genital reconstruction is irreversible and should clearly be undertaken only after an appropriate psychological evaluation. It is extremely important for all gender surgery that the surgeon has some professional relationship with the gender identity clinic service who refer the patient. The criteria for accepting such referrals are laid out in the *Standards of Care* published by the *World Professional Association for Transgender Health* (Currently, Coleman et al., 2012). Although at the time of writing, the current *Standards of Care* do not specifically mention non-binary surgery, it seems prudent to follow these guidelines for such patients as well; and no doubt future edition will include these patient groups.

In the case of non-binary individuals, it is vitally important to make sure that there is a complete understanding of what the patient actually wants. This may be a reconstruction resulting in genitalia which do not resemble either male or female; or which minimise certain aspects of male or female appearance, while overall resembling one or the other. A particular difficulty in this area can sometimes be patients who present for a 'cosmetic' procedure, but who have done so because they believe that they will not be able to get a referral for a procedure which delivers ambiguous or neutral genitalia. For this reason, it is the author's practice to ask younger patients who ask for a cosmetic operation if that is exactly what they want (older patients will often volunteer that they have opted for a cosmetic procedure because they wish to have a female appearance, but avoid the extra risks and maintenance which vaginoplasty entails). If there is any doubt in the surgeon's mind over exactly what surgery is requested, a conversation with the referring gender identity clinic service, or a request for a re-evaluation, would be appropriate.

Summary

* Non-binary 'surgeries' have been performed throughout history with varying degrees of success.
* It is vital to determine precisely what non-binary patients are requesting surgically and, if necessary, what they really want.
* Some non-binary patients may have endeavoured to perform self-surgery in desperation. These patients should be assisted surgically and, if necessary, psychologically.
* Birth-assigned males may opt for any of a variety of surgical options depending upon either their identity, the pragmatics of their situation, or both.
* As increasing numbers of such surgeries are performed, there may be some merit in general physicians having a basic familiarity with the anatomy so created.

References

Bellringer, J. (2007). Genital Surgery. In J. Barrett (Ed.), *Transsexualism and Other Disorders of Gender Identity* (pp. 209–219). Oxford: Radcliffe.
Coleman, E., Bockting, W., Botzer, M., Cohen-Kettenis, P., DeCuypere, G., Feldman, J., et al. (2012). Standards of Care for the Health of Transsexual,

Transgender, and Gender-Nonconforming people, Version 7. *International Journal of Transgenderism, 13*, 165–232.

Fang, R. H., Chen, C. F., & Ma, S. A. (1992). A New Method for Clitoroplasty in Male-to-Female Sex Reassignment Surgery. *Plastic and Reconstructive Surgery, 89*(4), 679–682.

Lawrence, A. A. (2006). Patient-Reported Complications and Functional Outcomes of Male-to-Female Sex Reassignment Surgery. *Archives of Sexual Behavior, 35*, 717–727.

Pinch, G. (2004). *Egyptian Mythology: A Guide to the Gods, Goddesses, and Traditions of Ancient Egypt.* New York: Oxford University Press.

Rubin, S. (1993). Sex Reassignment Surgery Male-to-Female. *Scandinavian Journal of Urology and Nephrology, 154*, S1–S28.

Scheidel, W. (2009). *Rome and China: Comparative Perspectives on Ancient World Empires.* New York: Oxford University Press.

Watanayusaki, S. (2015). *SRS Procedures. The Suporn Clinic.* Retrieved December 12, 2015, from http://www.supornclinic.com/restricted/SRS/SRSTechnique.aspx

Further Reading

Bellringer, J. (2007). Genital Surgery. In J. Barrett (Ed.), *Transsexualism and Other Disorders of Gender Identity* (pp. 209–219). Oxford: Radcliffe.

Coleman, E., Bockting, W., Botzer, M., Cohen-Kettenis, P., DeCuypere, G., Feldman, J., et al. (2012). Standards of Care for the Health of Transsexual, Transgender, and Gender-Nonconforming People, Version 7. *International Journal of Transgenderism, 13*, 165–232.

Richards, C., Bouman, W. P., Seal, L., Barker, M. J., Nieder, T., & T'Sjoen, G. (2016). Non-binary or Genderqueer Genders. *International Review of Psychiatry, 28*(1), 95–102.

13

Genital Surgery for Bodies Commonly Gendered as Female

David Ralph, Nim Christopher, and Giulio Garaffa

Introduction

Genital surgery for birth-assigned females undergoing gender reassignment generally consists of the following two broad groups of procedures:

Gynaecological procedures

- Hysterectomy
- Bilateral salpingo-oophorectomy
- Vaginectomy

D. Ralph • N. Christopher (✉) • G. Garaffa
St Peters Andrology Centre, London, UK

© The Author(s) 2017
C. Richards et al. (eds.), *Genderqueer and Non-Binary Genders*, Critical and Applied
Approaches in Sexuality, Gender and Identity, DOI 10.1057/978-1-137-51053-2_13

Total male genital reconstruction

- Metoidioplasty—converting a clitoris into a small penis (micropenis)
- Phalloplasty—standard size penis
- Urethroplasty
- Scrotoplasty
- Glans sculpting
- Clitoroplasty
- Testis prosthesis
- Penile prosthesis for vaginal or anal penetrative sex

There are very little accurate published data on the percentage of trans men that decide to undergo genital reconstructive surgery. This is in part due to patients transitioning in one country but then having the genital surgery in other countries. The true incidence of trans men is also unknown. The only reliable data available are the referral rates to Gender Identity Clinic services (GICs), which appear to grossly underestimate the incidence of trans men. Such genital surgery is relatively expensive and time consuming, and not all public health-care programmes will fund it; hence patients will go to other countries for surgery where it may be cheaper. Many surgical units performing such surgery have published neither their numbers nor where their patients come from. From a US survey of major surgical units in 2001, data were extrapolated that suggested a 5% metoidioplasty rate and 6% phalloplasty rate, giving a total of 11% genital surgery rate for trans men who were US residents (Horton, 2008). In the United Kingdom, the vast majority of trans men requesting genital surgery get referred to our centre. We estimate only about 10% of trans men being seen at GICs go on to have genital reconstructive surgery. This is based on a patient referral rate to GICs in the United Kingdom of about 250 per month in 2014 with a 2:1 ratio in favour of birth-assigned males (UK Trans Info, 2014) and our current rate of about 100 new phalloplasty or metoidioplasty operations per year. Historically, there were much higher referral rates for genital surgery for trans women. However, as referral rates for gender reassignment for people assigned male at birth and people assigned female at birth are now reaching parity (Kreukels et al., 2012; Zucker & Lawrence, 2009), and as knowledge and realistic expectations of the surgical creation of a penis (phalloplasty) are becoming more commonplace; this percentage will increase. The 2015 new referral rates to UK GICs have increased to over 400 new referrals per month (UK Trans Info, 2015), which will need a significant increase in resources for both GIC professionals and surgical capacity.

An increasing proportion of notionally trans men are falling into the grouping of non-binary gender. In part, some of this is due to patients labelling themselves as binary trans men in order to get referred for genital surgery from the GIC. However, once they are assessed in the surgical units, it becomes clear that what they want is a partial treatment request. As non-binary gender comprises a continuous spectrum from completely female to completely male, genital surgery requirements are accordingly very varied.

At the more 'male' end of the spectrum, a patient may request removal of all female internal and external genitalia and formation of penis with scrotum and testis prostheses and ability to void urine standing. Those with phalloplasty often request penile prosthesis to achieve rigidity for penetrative sexual intercourse. The phallus is usually reshaped with glans sculpting to give a circumcised appearance. Those having metoidioplasty can choose either a circumcised or uncircumcised appearance. Those having phalloplasty often have the clitoris buried under the skin to lose the female appearance, but still preserve sexual function (Garcia, Christopher, Luca, Spilotros, & Ralph, 2014).

Natally assigned female non-binary people may opt for this approach if it accords with their identity or, more commonly, one of a variety of other approaches detailed below. There is no discrete diagnostic category, and patients give varying reasons for the partial surgical treatment choices they make (Beek, Kreukels, Cohen-Kettenis, & Steensma, 2016). The various genital surgical procedures and modifications for natally assigned female non-binary patients are therefore discussed below in the context of surgeries for trans men.

Genital Surgery Requirements

All patients will have been referred from a GIC having complied with the World Professional Association for Transgender Health (WPATH) standards of care for genital surgery (Coleman et al., 2012). For the gynaecological surgery, the following six criteria are required:

1. Persistent, well-documented gender dysphoria;
2. Capacity to make a fully informed decision and to consent for treatment;
3. Age of majority in a given country;
4. If significant medical or mental health concerns are present, they must be well controlled;
5. Twelve continuous months of hormone therapy as appropriate to the patient's gender goals (unless hormones are not clinically indicated for the individual). For genital reconstructive surgery, an extra criterion is also required;
6. Twelve continuous months of living in a gender role that is congruent with their gender identity;

Both types of surgery need recommendations from two GIC professionals that they are ready for genital reconstruction surgery.

All patients must have stopped smoking for a minimum of 6 months prior to genital reconstructive surgery. Smoking is the single biggest factor resulting in phallus loss and poor healing of skin grafts. For patients who are on nicotine replacement including E-cigarettes, we recommend stopping 1 month prior to surgery and they may restart 1 month afterwards. In the long term, smokers have a higher rate of urethral strictures than non-smokers in cisgender men undergoing urethroplasty (Breyer et al., 2010; Sinha, Singh, & Sankhwar, 2010), and there is no reason why this should be any better in trans men with a totally reconstructed urethra, so it is best to quit smoking for good.

Our weight criterion is a body mass index (BMI) of 30 or less for phalloplasty. For metoidioplasty, cosmetic and functional results are better, the thinner the patient; so a lower BMI is desirable. Overweight patients are more likely to have haematoma, which can compromise the blood supply of the phallus, and often need a bigger flap of tissue to make the phallus. This bigger flap may be prone to necrosis at the edges if it is too big for the blood supply.

Hair in the neo-urethra leads to a lifetime of surgical intervention for complications, so it is best to use non-hairy skin. If the patient needs hair removal for the urethral segment, then this may take 6–12 months to achieve via electrolysis or laser hair removal. We also recommend waiting a further 3 months after the hair removal is finished to ensure no late hair growth before making the neo-urethra. We often see patients for an assessment prior to their official GIC referral for genital surgery so that the weight loss, stopping smoking, and hair removal can be completed before they are officially referred so as to avoid unnecessary delays in their pathway. It is important to give these patients realistic expectations of the cosmetic and functional outcomes of genital surgery. We also emphasise the multiple procedures and post-operative recovery times required to achieve the desired outcome, and if there are complications, then extra surgery may be needed.

Gynaecological Procedures

Hysterectomy and bilateral oophorectomy are preferably performed laparoscopically to ensure minimal morbidity. If a skin incision is needed, then a lower abdominal midline incision does not preclude any form of future phalloplasty or metoidioplasty (the creation of a smaller penis from the clitoris). A transverse or Pfannenstiel incision results in a significant compromise of a future pubic phalloplasty (PP) due to interference with the blood supply to the potential skin flap. Related to these procedures, non-binary patients have requested the following:

"I want to keep the cervix for sexual sensation…"

"I'd like to keep the ovaries for bone protection…"

"I'm considering keeping my ovaries to possibly have eggs for IVF in future…"

"I don't really feel the need to have the uterus removed and am happy to have regular cervical screening and ultrasound assessments…"

The commonest technique to remove the uterus is laparoscopically assisted vaginal hysterectomy. The pelvis is accessed via three abdominal ports. The uterine and ovarian pedicles are divided and mobilised from inside, following which the cervix is mobilised transvaginally before removing the uterus, fallopian tubes, and ovaries transvaginally. The vaginal vault can be closed from above or below. It is possible to do this completely laparoscopically using a power morcellator to mince the uterus for easy removal via one of the laparoscopic ports. However, this method has been strongly discouraged by the Food and Drug Administration in the United States due to the potential risk of disseminating an undiagnosed uterine sarcoma (U.S. Food and Drug Administration, 2014).

A subtotal hysterectomy leaves the cervix intact and attached to the vagina. The uterus would need to be removed via an enlarged port incision usually at the umbilicus. If an ovary is requested to be left in situ, then usually just one is removed for easier monitoring. In our experience, nearly every patient who requested this eventually asked for the remaining ovary to be removed. Gynaecological cancer risk is low in the trans men group and usually the uterus is very small (Wierckx et al., 2010). Large fibroids are more common in patients transitioning in older age groups and may necessitate open surgery rather than laparoscopic.

Vaginectomy for trans men can be performed via a number of different muscle-preserving techniques. This is usually offered as a mucosal vaginectomy as opposed to a radical vaginectomy, where all the muscles are removed as well, which is an operation for vaginal cancer. The mucosa is the sole source of vaginal secretions, and removal or destruction of the mucosa results in cessation of secretions, which is what most trans men desire. Mucosal excision is straightforward in the outer half of the vagina but problematic in the deeper portions because of strong adherence to the vaginal musculature. As a result, significant bleeding from the paravaginal venous plexuses can be a problem if large parts of the muscular layer are also removed. The mucosa can be excised using blunt dissection, sharp dissection, laser, diathermy, or theoretically high-pressure water jet technology. The idea is to minimise bleeding and risk of perforation of nearby structures such as bladder, urethra, or rectum.

Our preferred technique in the United Kingdom since 2012, as the only major centre providing Genital Reconstruction Surgery (GRS) for trans men, is ablation vaginectomy using cut electrocautery on a high-power setting with a rollerball electrode to vaporise the mucosa leaving the muscular layer intact. There is almost no bleeding with the ablation method and also very little risk of perforation of bladder, urethra, or rectum. Residual vaginal mucosa can give rise to cyst formation in the vaginal space, but this is easily dealt with by re-ablation or re-excision. Once the introitus is closed externally, it will take a few months for the vaginal space to obliterate. Occasionally, incomplete removal of Bartholin's glands in the introitus can give rise to external cysts, which are easily removed.

At least one centre in the United States also offers closure of the vaginal introitus, whilst leaving the vaginal mucosa intact. The vaginal vault is left open to allow vaginal secretions to drain into the peritoneal cavity where they can be reabsorbed. Theoretically, bowel can fall into the vaginal space as in an internal hernia, which may cause problems such as intermittent bowel obstruction.

Whatever method of vaginectomy is performed, the introitus is closed in such a way as to form a male perineum with a flat area between anus and bottom of the scrotum. This also allows the labia majora to be conjoined into one scrotal sac to reduce the bifid appearance otherwise. Obviously, vaginectomy can only be offered if hysterectomy and removal of cervix has been performed first. Related to these procedures, non-binary patients have requested the following:

"My main sexual sensation is around the vaginal opening so I'd like to preserve that…"

A patient who was in a relationship with a man stated:

"I'd like to keep the vagina for penetrative sex as otherwise my only other option is anal sex…"

A bisexual patient stated:

"I need a big penis and need to keep the vagina to satisfy both my partners…"

It is not a problem to leave the vagina and introitus completely intact for sexual penetration. The main issue arises when the patient is also requesting an urethroplasty to void from the tip of phallus or metoidioplasty. Because a small flap of vaginal mucosa is used to create the bottom portion of neo-urethra and extra tissue is needed to protect the urethroplasty; the vaginal introitus is usually narrowed during the skin closure and patients are advised that they will need to self-dilate the vaginal opening once the urethra has healed. For those patients who do not wish to retain the ability to be penetrated vaginally, the introitus is deliberately narrowed to allow secretions to drain, but allow an inconspicuous appearance.

Total Genital Reconstruction

Metoidioplasty is the formation of a micropenis from the enlarged clitoris after testosterone stimulation (Djordjevic & Bizic, 2013). Scrotoplasty and mons fat excision are often performed concurrently in order to remove bulk from around the base of the micropenis to make it appear larger. If voiding from the tip of the micropenis is required, then an urethroplasty is also needed, although some patients are happy to void sitting. For trans men, this can be performed in one, two, or three stages depending upon the surgical unit.

Because the clitoris always points downwards, it is necessary to divide the 'urethral plate' in most cases unless there is significant clitoral hypertrophy. The 'urethral plate' is the pink tissue between the glans and native urethral meatus. Once this is divided, the micropenis can be pulled up with an increase in length of 2–3 cm on average. If no urethral extension is required, then the labia minora skin is merely wrapped around the clitoral shaft to reconstitute the body of the micropenis. Some surgeons also divide the clitoral suspensory ligament, which attaches dorsally to the pubic bone for extra length, but doing this makes the clitoris fall forward and downwards away from the pubis.

If voiding from the tip is desired, then usually a buccal mucosa graft is placed on the divided 'urethral plate' to form the future urethral back wall. In one-stage procedures, a labia minora flap is used to form the front wall of the urethra immediately. In multi-stage procedures, the buccal graft is left to mature first (to confirm no further shrinkage) for 6 months before tubularisation to form the neo-urethra. If the patient is happy to void sitting, then the native urethral meatus is extended a couple of centimetres to a new opening at the bottom of the scrotum in an unobtrusive position. For those voiding from the tip, the head of the micropenis usually will not be long enough to be able to stretch it clearly past the zip/fly of their trousers, and so may create some difficulties with voiding standing up. However with careful manipulation, it should be possible to direct the urinary stream so that it doesn't splash onto the clothing.

The upper portions of the labia majora extend above the base of the micropenis so these are mobilised, sometimes with a VY-plasty technique, to bring this area below the base of the micropenis. This then forms the scrotum. Best functional and visual results are with a concurrent vaginectomy as this then avoids a bifid appearance. Mons fat can be excised via the upper labial incisions or from a transverse pubic incision or a mini-abdominoplasty as needed. Some centres insert small testicular prostheses simultaneously, and some put them in at a separate second or third stage. Some patients are happy with the scrotal appearance just with the fat content and never request testicular prostheses. In some cases, the round ligaments or labial fat can be incorporated into the micropenis shaft for bulk.

Related to metoidioplasty, non-binary patients have requested the following:

"I just want a clitoral release and removal of the flaps (labia minora)..."

"I don't really want any scrotum so please remove it and make as flat as possible and leave the clitoris alone..."

Performing a clitoral release and removal of labia minora is very simple, but the scrotum will be bifid and start above the base of micropenis. Removal of just the labia minora and majora is again very simple to do, but patients must be advised that if they are very thin, there will be no padding around the urethral meatus. This can result in the sensitive pink introitus tissue always being in contact with clothing when sitting which may be very uncomfortable.

In contrast to metoidioplasty, full-size phalloplasty requires sufficient skin and subcutaneous fat to tubularise into an usual size phallus. There are essentially two types of donor site depending on the blood supply:

* Blood supply is via the skin and connective tissue (local flap)
  * PP
  * Extended groin (EG) flap
  * Gilles flap
  * Many others

* Blood supply is via a dedicated artery and vein(s) (free flap)
  * Radial artery phalloplasty
  * Antero-lateral thigh (ALT) flap
  * Musculocutaneous latissimus dorsi (MLD) flap
  * Gracilis flap (GF)
  * Many others

In most patients, a block of skin and subcutaneous fat of 14 cm length by 12–13 cm width is used for the new phallus. Once this is tubularised, the final size depends on the elasticity of the skin and weight of the fat. If the skin is elastic and the fat heavy, then it will become bigger than the initial dimensions. If the converse, then the phallus will collapse to a smaller size. Thus, it is important to ask the patient to get to an appropriate weight such that there is sufficient fatty tissue, but not too much to get the desired result. Our surgical criterion is a BMI of 18–30. Thus, there is significant natural variation in the final phallus dimensions once it is made. If a neo-urethra is also required, then another 4–5 cm width of tissue is required. We always ask the patients to discuss the girth of the phallus, once it has been made, with their partners in case it will need to be narrowed down before a penile prosthesis is inserted.

Phalloplasty is a multi-stage procedure. The minimum number of operations is two. The first being to make the phallus, urethra, scrotum, and glans, and the second being to insert penile and testicular prosthesis. Penile prosthesis insertion is normally delayed until there is some protective phallus sensation. Our practice is to use three operations. The first being to make the phallus; the second is to complete the urethra, glans, and scrotum; and the third is to insert penile and testicular prosthesis. Our rationale is shorter hospital stay for the first operation as no urine is going through the freshly made phallus, and we believe that the glans sculpting looks much better when done at a separate stage to the phallus. Other techniques may require more stages than this.

A PP is constructed by cutting three sides of a rectangular local flap with the base (notional blood supply) centred at the top of the clitoral fold at the pubis. This is then tubularised to form the phallus. The resulting abdominal defect is closed with rotation skin flaps resulting in a long horizontal lower abdominal scar that is easily hidden by the underpants. This type of phalloplasty has no protective or erogenous sensation in the distal portion and normal sensation in the base.

The EG flap is based on the circumflex iliac vessels and a de-epithelialised strip of tissue near the groin to elongate the pedicle of the base of the flap. The visible skin component stretches out sideways over the iliac crest. The de-epithelialised portion allows the base of the phallus to be tunnelled under the groin skin to the pubic area to be sited correctly. Often this gives rise to a very bulky pedicle under the skin on the side of the donor site. This works better in children and adolescents as their skin is not hairy and less fat (Perovic, 1995). The donor defect can be closed primarily but may need skin grafting. There is no sensation in this flap. It also preserves the forearm for use if they need a better phalloplasty once they reach adult age.

We normally only use the Gilles flap as a salvage procedure when other free flap phalloplasties have failed and there are no other options available (Gilles & Harrison, 1948). A suitcase handle-type pedicle is created in the non-hairy 'love handles' area of the side of the abdomen, with the blood supply coming from both sides of the pedicles. Using a delayed pedicle transfer technique, the base of the handle furthest away is transferred to the pubic area. Once the new blood supply is established, the other end is detached leaving the phallus hanging in the correct position from the pubic area. This requires multiple small operations and has the risk of pedicle necrosis if the blood supply is inadequate at any time. There is no protective or erogenous sensation with this phalloplasty. It is possible to make an integrated neo-urethra with the EG and Gilles flaps (if there is sufficient non-hairy skin), but the urethral blood supply is totally dependent on the phallus. If there is disruption of the blood supply of the phallus for any reason, commonly phallus dilatation during insertion of penile prosthesis or a penile prosthesis infection, then the urethra is the first thing to become ischaemic and stricture down.

Free flaps are much more successful than local flaps because of the dedicated blood supply. They are particularly suited for neo-urethral formation as they are more resistant to shrinkage. By definition, a free flap involves disconnecting the flap from the donor site and using microsurgical techniques to re-anastomose the vessels and nerves to the recipient site. Some free flaps have sufficiently long vessels that they can be used as pedicled flaps, that is, without disconnecting. These can include the ALT flaps and GCs. The only donor sites where sufficient tissue can be taken for both phallus and neo-urethra together are the radial forearm and ALT flaps.

Because so much tissue is needed, donor site morbidity and cosmetic appearance are a significant consideration for patients. The donor site would need to be covered with a skin graft. Care would be taken to use the most cosmetic skin graft for visible donor sites like the forearm. If a neo-urethra is being planned, then a tube in tube technique would be used, for example, for radial forearm or ALT (Chang & Hwang, 1984; Felici & Felici, 2006). Here, the 3–4 cm width urethral part is tubed with the skin on the inside and then the larger phallus portion is wrapped around it with the skin on the outside. All other phalloplasties would need the urethra to be made from the forearm separately as a radial forearm flap urethroplasty, which leaves a much smaller cosmetic defect on the forearm. The MLD flap in particular is able to allow the use of buccal or skin graft onto the muscle component, which takes well, and this can then be tubularised at a later date to form the neo-urethra (Perovic, Djinovic, Bumbasirevic, Djordjevic, & Vukovic 2007). The scrotal portion of the neo-urethra is made with labia minora and the existing 'urethral plate' of the clitoris and a small anterior vaginal mucosa flap at the bottom end. This vaginal flap incorporates Skene's glands (para-urethral glands) into the neo-urethra. This allows some patients the ability to have a pseudo-ejaculate when they are sexually excited. Skene's glands are homologous to the prostate in cisgender males and can produce large amounts of fluid during 'female orgasm', which is similar in composition to prostatic fluid (Wimpissinger, Stifter, Grin, & Stackl, 2007). They are not always present and have been thought to be the cause of 'female ejaculation' in some cisgender females (Pastor, 2013).

Scrotoplasty is different from metoidioplasty in that the base of phallus is above the top of the labia majora so the lower labia majora are rotated or pushed upwards to form the scrotal sac. Again, best cosmetic results are when a vaginectomy is also performed, as this reduces the bifid appearance of the scrotum.

Glans sculpting can be done at the same time as the phalloplasty procedure or at a separate stage. A distally based skin flap is rolled up to form the coronal ridge. A skin graft is used to cover the exposed fat to form the coronal sulcus. Because all skin grafts contract as they heal, this allows the formation of a shaft, narrower neck, and prominent head or glans. This is the basis of the Norfolk technique. Other methods involve taking extra skin distally in the phalloplasty flap and using this to form the glans at the same time as the phallus—the so-called cricket bat transformer flap. This can be made from the forearm or MLD flaps which have enough spare skin and results in no suture line at the urethral meatus (Gottlieb & Levine, 1993). The only downside is that the length of the phallus is smaller unless extra skin is also incorporated, which is not always possible.

Clitoroplasty involves repositioning the clitoris to a different location without interfering with sexual sensation too much (Garcia et al., 2014). In our centre, most patients ask for it to be not visible, that is, buried just under the dermis of the skin near the base of the phallus. This allows for sexual stimulation during intercourse. Additionally, if a penile prosthesis is inserted later, it will theoretically push the buried clitoris against the skin from the inside giving extra stimulation. Some are happy to leave it exactly where it is on the outside, but of course, this will result in a bifid scrotum. Some centres mobilise the clitoris with the urethral plate and position it on the pubic bone as part of the urethroplasty, so it is under the phallus. For flaps that come with cutaneous nerves, for example, radial forearm, ALT, and MLD, it is routine to connect one of the clitoral nerves to the flap nerve to allow sexual sensation on the phallus eventually. The other flap nerves are connected usually to the ilio-inguinal or genito-femoral nerves for touch sensation. Touch and sexual sensation has been reported to be successful in 90% of cases after 2-year follow-up (Doornaert et al., 2011; Garaffa, Christopher, & Ralph, 2010). Anecdotally, some patients in our clinic have reported the ability to reach orgasm from only phallic stimulation. Clitoral repositioning is usually done at the same time as scrotoplasty and urethroplasty.

There are fewer variations for non-binary patients in full-size phalloplasty. Some typical requests are:

"I just want something small to pee from that is bigger than a metoidioplasty and I'm not bothered about having sex…"

"I'll have a forearm phalloplasty as it looks nice but don't connect the urethra as I don't want problems peeing…"

"I need a pant-filler so I can take my grandson swimming without getting embarrassed…"

"I'm happy with the phallus as it is and don't want glans sculpting…"

A forearm flap taken from the distal part of the forearm of about 8–9 cm in length can be tubularised to form a shorter phallus; and if less width of tissue is taken, then the phallus can be narrower. However, it would be impossible to insert a penile prosthesis later, although the donor defect would be much smaller. This gives a phallus big enough to hold to pass urine, but not longer than 8–9 cm. This will be long enough to easily pull out past the zip/fly of their trousers when passing urine standing.

A fully reconstructed neo-urethra has two problems inherent in the design. The first is spraying of urine due to turbulent flow along the urethra, which occurs in varying degrees in all patients. The second is post void dribbling (PVD) due to the absence of a functional bulbospongiosus muscle around the scrotal part of the neo-urethra to squeeze the last few drops out. This problem also happens in natal males if this muscle stops working. PVD is variable and occurs in up to 70% of patients. Unlike the phallic neo-urethra, the scrotal neo-urethra is made of thinner and stretchier skin and can balloon out with time and allow more urine to be retained after voiding. If severe, and assuming there is no distal urethral stricture, the only solution is to revise the baggy scrotal neo-urethra to narrow it down so that less urine can collect to dribble later. Those patients who request the urethra not to be connected, but want a forearm flap, have the lower end of the neo-urethra just next to the clitoris but void through the native meatus lower down. This does mean that the neo-urethra can be connected at any time in the future should they change their mind. The easiest way to make a pant-filler is with a PP as all the scars are low down and easily covered with shorts, underpants, or swimming trunks.

Testicular prosthesis can be made of liquid silicone, solid gel silicone, or saline. Saline-filled testis prosthesis is the only permissible option in the United States. In Europe, solid gel silicone testes are used most often. The solid gel testes are rupture resistant and usually will last a lifetime and have varying textures depending on the brand. Liquid silicone testes are much softer but are prone to rupture like the saline-filled testis and so will need replacing when broken. Some units use a permanently implanted tissue expander testis (Osmed™), which is easily implanted as a 3-ml volume device into the scrotum. This absorbs fluid from the surrounding tissues gradually to the maximum volume of about 30 ml over a few weeks.

Erectile devices are needed by the majority of patients that want to engage in penetrative sex with their phallus. Some pubic phalloplasties have sufficiently dense fat that penetration can be achieved with just a condom to compact the fat a little more. However, the fat does become softer with time. For those who wish them, there are two types of penile prosthesis: inflatable, or malleable/semi-rigid. The semi-rigid prosthesis has a metallic core covered with a silicone outer sheath, which allows the rigidity and bendability for concealment. They last a very long time, but are more prone to erosion of the phallus due to the stiffness. Inflatable devices usually have three components; reservoir, pump, and cylinders—and utilise a hydraulic system where the pump replaces the second testicle. The reservoir is placed in the abdomen and the cylinder(s) in the phallus. The pump is a two-way control valve putting fluid into the cylinder for the erection and pumping it out back to the reservoir for flaccidity. This is more physiological and has less risk of erosion, as the device is flaccid most of the time. Unfortunately, because it uses moving parts, it is more prone to mechanical failure than the semi-rigid devices. As with all prosthetic devices, the risk of infection is high and has been reported as high as 11.9% (Hoebeke et al., 2010). Because there is less protection for the device in a neo-phallus, it is more prone to mechanical failure than in cisgender males and about 50% of devices are explanted or exchanged after 6–10 years (Hoebeke et al., 2010). The addition of a Dacron™ sheath (woven polyethylene terephthalate—a synthetic polyester fabric) or similar material to protect the device improves durability, but also increases infection rates.

Non-binary patients who request penile prosthesis usually will have wanted to retain the vagina for additional sexual function. They will often not take the risk of added infection and multiple prosthesis revision surgery in the future. In addition, patients also use external strap-on devices for penetrative sex and those that do usually request a slightly smaller phallus so that it fits inside the device.

Summary

In summary, there are quite a few variations of the standard techniques that are applicable to the non-binary person assigned female at birth. These are relatively straightforward to perform. Surgeons and GIC professionals should be aware of these variations when referring for genital surgery.

References

Beek, T. F., Kreukels, B. P. C., Cohen-Kettenis, P. T., & Steensma, T. D. (2016). Partial Treatment Requests and Underlying Motives of Applicants for Gender Affirming Interventions. *Journal of Sexual Medicine, 12*(11), 2201–2205.

Breyer, B., McAninch, J., Whitson, J., Eisenberg, M., Mehdizadeh, J., Myers, J., et al. (2010). Multivariate Analysis of Risk Factors for Long-Term Urethroplasty Outcome. *Journal of Urology, 183*(2), 613–617.

Chang, T., & Hwang, W. (1984). Forearm Flap in One-Stage Reconstruction of the Penis. *Plastic and Reconstructive Surgery, 74*(2), 251–258.

Coleman, E., Bockting, W., Botzer, M., Cohen-Kettenis, P., DeCuypere, G., Feldman, J., et al. (2012). Standards of Care for the health of Transsexual, Transgender, and Gender-Nonconforming People, Version 7. *International Journal of Transgenderism, 13*, 165–232.

Djordjevic, M., & Bizic, M. (2013). Comparison of Two Different Methods for Urethral Lengthening in Female to Male (Metoidioplasty) Surgery. *The Journal of Sexual Medicine, 10*(5), 1431–1438.

Doornaert, M., Hoebeke, P., Ceulemans, P., T'Sjoen, G., Heylens, G., & Monstrey, S. (2011). Penile Reconstruction with the Radial Forearm Flap: An Update. *Handchirurgie, Mikrochirurgie, plastische Chirurgie, 43*(4), 208–214.

Felici, N., & Felici, A. (2006). A New Phalloplasty Technique: The Free Anterolateral Thigh Flap Phalloplasty. *Journal of Plastic, Reconstructive & Aesthetic Surgery, 59*(2), 153–157.

Garaffa, G., Christopher, N., & Ralph, D. (2010). Total Phallic Reconstruction in Female to Male Transsexuals. *European Urology, 57*(4), 715–722.

Garcia, M., Christopher, N., Luca, F., Spilotros, M., & Ralph, D. (2014). Overall Satisfaction, Sexual Function, and the Durability of Neophallus Dimensions Following Staged Female to Male Genital Gender Confirming Surgery: The Institute of Urology, London U.K. Experience. *Translational Andrology and Urology, 3*(2), 156–162. Retrieved from http://www.amepc.org/tau/article/view/3748

Gillies, H., & Harrison, R. (1948). Congenital Absence of the Penis with Embryological Considerations. *British Journal of Plastic Surgery, 1*, 8–28.

Gottlieb, L., & Levine, L. (1993). A New Design for the Radial Forearm Free-flap Phallic Construction. *Plastic and Reconstructive Surgery, 92*(2), 276–283.

Hoebeke, P., Decaestecker, K., Beysens, M., Opdenakker, Y., Lumen, N., & Monstrey, S. (2010). Erectile Implants in Female-to-Male Transsexuals: Our Experience in 129 Patients. *European Urology, 57*(2), 334–340.

Horton, M. (2008, September). *The Prevalence of SRS Among US Residents, Out & Equal Workplace Summit*. Retrieved from http://www.tgender.net/taw/thbcost.html#prevalence

Kreukels, B., Haraldsen, I., De Cuypere, G., Richter-Appelt, H., Gijs, L., & Cohen-Kettenis, P. (2012). A European Network for the Investigation of Gender Incongruence: The ENIGI Initiative. *European Psychiatry, 27*, 445–450.

Pastor, Z. (2013). Female Ejaculation Orgasm Vs. Coital Incontinence: A Systematic Review. *Journal of Sexual Medicine, 10*(7), 1682–1691.

Perovic, S. (1995). Phalloplasty in Children and Adolescents Using the Extended Pedicle Island Groin Flap. *Journal of Urology, 154*(2 Pt 2), 848–853.

Perovic, S., Djinovic, R., Bumbasirevic, M., Djordjevic, M., & Vukovic, P. (2007). Total Phalloplasty Using a Musculocutaneous Latissimus Dorsi Flap. *BJU International, 100*(4), 899–905.

Sinha, R., Singh, V., & Sankhwar, S. (2010). Does Tobacco Consumption Influence Outcome of Oral Mucosa Graft Urethroplasty? *Urology Journal, 7*(1), 45–50.

U.S. Food and Drug Administration. (2014, November 24). *Update Laparoscopic Uterine Power Morcellation in Hysterectomy and Myomectomy: FDA Safety Communication*. Retrieved from http://www.fda.gov/MedicalDevices/Safety/AlertsandNotices/ucm424443.htm

UK Trans Info. (2014). *Current Waiting Times and Patient Population for Gender Identity Services in the UK*. Retrieved from http://uktrans.info/attachments/article/341/PatientPopulationSept14.pdf

UK Trans Info. (2015). *Current Waiting Times and Patient Population for Gender Identity Services in the UK*. Retrieved from http://uktrans.info/attachments/article/341/patientpopulation-july15.pdf

Wierckx, K., Mueller, S., Weyers, S., Caenegem, E., Roef, G., Heylens, G., et al. (2010). Long-Term Evaluation of Cross-Sex Hormone Treatment in Transsexual Persons. *The Journal of Sexual Medicine, 9*(10), 2641–2651.

Wimpissinger, F., Stifter, K., Grin, W., & Stackl, W. (2007). The Female Prostate Revisited: Perineal Ultrasound and Biochemical Studies of Female Ejaculate. *The Journal of Sexual Medicine, 4*(5), 1388–1393.

Zucker, K., & Lawrence, A. (2009). Epidemiology of Gender Identity Disorder: Recommendations for the Standards of Care of the World Professional Association for Transgender Health. *International Journal of Transgenderism, 11*, 8–18.

14

Future Directions

Alex Iantaffi

Introduction

Every time I approached this chapter, I found myself in a freeze reaction at the realisation of the task undertaken: to write a chapter on the future directions of non-binary genders. If you have read the book in its entirety, I hope that you will be understanding the enormity of this enterprise and forgiving the shortcomings of this chapter. If you have not yet read the rest of the book, I will not judge you, but rather invite you to do so, as there is an astounding amount of knowledge and expertise within the covers of this book. For those readers in the latter category, I use the expression *non-binary genders* to indicate any gender identities that do not fall under the polarised dichotomy of male or female. I use the term *cis* to indicate identities where sex assigned at birth and gender identity align, and *trans* for those identities where those two constructs do not align. I know I am keeping my definitions

A. Iantaffi (✉)
University of Minnesota, Minneapolis, MN, USA

© The Author(s) 2017
C. Richards et al. (eds.), *Genderqueer and Non-Binary Genders*, Critical and Applied Approaches in Sexuality, Gender and Identity, DOI 10.1057/978-1-137-51053-2_14

fairly simple, whereas those identities and experiences are far more complex and nuanced. I hope that by maintaining some initial, simple definitions, I might keep the landscape of our journey into the future directions of non-binary genders as broad as possible.

In this chapter, I attempt to explore some of the potential impacts of non-binary genders on a range of disciplines as well as on White Western minority cultures. In some ways, this feels like a fool's journey, given that predicting the future is always an uncertain business. However, I invite you to embrace the quality of fool with me: that is, an openness to new possibilities, the willingness to move into the unknown, the courage to begin the journey without knowing its destination, and the wonder of the path unfolding as we go. I also invite you to broaden your horizons, given that it is impossible, in my opinion, to consider the future directions of non-binary genders without also addressing the movement towards decolonisation of identities and experiences (Arvin, Tuck & Morrill, 2013) increasingly acknowledged within public discourse; The impact of feminist science (Wyer, Barbercheck, Cookmeyer, Ozturk, & Wayne, 2013); And our general understanding of identities, experiences, and communities as intersectional (Cho, Crenshaw & McCall, 2013; Crenshaw, 1991) and therefore essentially not easily dissectible in neat, categorical constructs.

Intersectionality—named by Kimberlé Crenshaw (Crenshaw, 1991)—is the study of the inextricable and intersecting dynamics of power and oppression, often resulting in experiences of discrimination that cannot easily be attributed to a single identity category. In this chapter, I invite you to consider non-binary genders, not as a single umbrella category, but rather as just one axis within complex shapes of experiences and identities, not fixed in time and space. Informed by positioning theory (Harré & Van Langenhove, 1998)—that is the idea that we are continuously invited and inviting ourselves and others into a range of dynamic locations within a complex web of relational and power systems—I approach the future directions of non-binary genders in this chapter, as a fluid dance between I, as author, you as readers, and the multiple positions and systems we find ourselves in, at the moment of our fleeting encounters. On this esoteric sounding note, let's be done with introductions and maps, as you have already been informed they might be of little use on this journey, and let's begin to speculate the trajectories of non-binary genders. I conclude our journey, and the chapter, with a bullet point summary of some of the main ideas explored and some suggestions for further reading.

Identity Labels and Politics

Non-binary genders include a variety of labels (Richards et al., 2016) as detailed in earlier chapters in this book. Those labels are currently often grouped under the broader trans umbrella. This inclusion is both troubled and troublesome. It is troubled in that many individuals with non-binary identities and experience discuss not feeling 'trans enough', for not complying to trans normative narratives under this large umbrella term (Currah, 2006). It is troublesome as it blurs the lines between trans and cis identities and expressions. Who gets to decide the legitimacy of someone's trans identity? In the past, when seeking medical and legal transition-related services and acknowledgements, trans people often had to prove conformity to the gender binary in a range of ways, including adherence to heteronormativity through divorce and even sterilisation (Iantaffi, 2015; Irving, 2008). At the time of writing this chapter, this is no longer the case in many countries, yet trans people often feel that their gender identity might not be seen as legitimate if they do not conform to binary expectations of masculinity and femininity (Iantaffi & Bockting, 2011). Some trans people, of course, just want to live their lives (Richards, Barker, Lenihan, & Iantaffi, 2014), as well as not being magically exempt from the extensive influence that structural cisgenderism has on all of us. Increasingly, though, trans people are globally demanding the same choices available to most cis people: To live life on their own terms, and to express their gender identities and roles in a way that is coherent with other aspects of identities and larger value and belief systems. For example, some young trans feminine people want to be recognised as girls even when they choose to cut their hair short, be proud of their strength, not wear make-up or stereotypically feminine attire. There is also increased recognition that trans people have a broad range of sexual orientations (Iantaffi & Bockting, 2011), which are not to be seen as pathological or as negating the legitimacy of their gendered identities.

Among these communities and individuals, there are many who identify with non-binary genders. Further, several writers and activists are inviting more critical, racially informed, intersectional analyses of gender that challenge the universality of trans experiences, and even the construct of trans as an umbrella category (Boellstorff et al., 2014; Dutta & Roy, 2014; Lamble, 2008). Many indigenous and global activists, and scholars continue to remind us that non-binary genders, queer, and trans identities are not only not new, or innovative, but rather a result of the need to reclaim a broader range of gender and sexual diversity exterminated by colonisation and Christianisation (Robinson, 2012). In these contexts, gender is no longer a singular category that can be easily polarised, with non-binary genders being the fluid, movable fulcrum of balance; but rather a point of reference among others—a system that necessarily intersects with other systems, such as race and ethnicity, indigeneity, class, disability, age, religion, and citizenship. Within a systemic and intersectional analysis of gender, knowing someone's gender identity, expression, or role alone, without knowing also the other localities of their lived experiences, has little to no value, like a two-dimensional view in a three-dimensional world. Gender then becomes but one point in an interactive map, where the landscape is not fixed.

Within this analysis, labels, which usually distinguish between this and that, me and other, begin to blur, and identity politics increase in complexity. There can be no oppression Olympics, even though we can still map the most impacted by looking at disparities in education, health, employment, and socioeconomic status. And the current map indicates that some of the starkest disparities are being experienced in the liminal spaces of identities that do not fit neatly in normative paradigms (Harrison, Grant, & Herman, 2012), and on indigenous bodies that have already borne, and continue to bear, the impact of genocide (King, Smith, & Gracey, 2009). Nevertheless, the complexity of identity politics increases as our understanding of intersectionality becomes better understood in mainstream discourses.

In the USA in particular, there currently seems to be the desire to proudly affirm one's individual identity, as exemplified in one of the analyses looking at labels in a large survey of trans respondents, where 860 out of over 6000 respondents wrote in their own gender identity terms (Harrison et al., 2012), which could potentially be seen as stemming from a culture of rugged individualism. At the same time, there is a movement towards talking about the transgender community as monolithic, as exemplified by the Time article entitled *The Transgender Tipping Point* (Steinmetz, 2014). Within activism, in the same geographical contexts, there has been a call for trans people of colour to be heard; and especially trans feminine people of colour. The contrast between more public figures, such as the African-American actress Laverne Cox, or White athlete and socialite Caitlyn Jenner, and the lived experiences of less well-known trans feminine people, and especially people of colour in the USA, is vast.

While some could argue that celebrities bring increased visibility, and ultimately acceptance, for all, in reality, the intersection of socioeconomic status, race, education, citizenship, disability, and gender are still largely ignored or downplayed in mainstream media—including the potential risk that higher visibility might entail for many people, especially those who identifies as non-binary. In a mainstream culture that seemingly celebrates authenticity, people with non-binary identities and expressions are often most vulnerable to violence when at their most authentic, as pointed out by the artistic duo Darkmatter (http://www.darkmatterpoetry.com/). Therefore, in the area of identity labels and politics, one of the potential future directions of non-binary gender identities seems to trouble the liberal—and somewhat self-congratulatory—Anglo acceptance of trans bodies by inviting us to truly dismantle cisgenderism; to question the assumed essentialism of masculinity and femininity as natural polarities; to consider our complex, intersectional bodies and lived experiences; and to engage with a different framework of genders altogether.

Structural Repercussions

The potential structural repercussions of engaging with a non-binary, as well as potentially a non-Anglo, model of gender(s) are vast. Given the historical dominance of medical professionals over trans bodies, let us first consider what is happening in this arena. Non-binary genders are somewhat acknowledged in the newer *Standards of Care* of the *World Professional Association for Transgender Health* (Coleman et al., 2012). However, the implementation of these guidelines is still heavily influenced by cisgenderism and a binary understanding of gender. For example, there is still a burden of proof on trans people when dealing with health providers who need to produce letters or approve medical prescriptions. Trans people might still face varying levels of gatekeeping when seeking to modify their own body medically through hormonal or surgical interventions. Access to chosen healthcare providers, and the level of gatekeeping that might be faced, can vary greatly from country to country, and depending on whether the person seeking medical interventions is considered to be a minor or an adult. Proving one's gender identity, and the need for services, is particularly challenging for openly non-binary identified people, given that often conforming to an identity not aligned with one's sex assigned at birth, over a long period of time, is what professionals are looking for. This is particularly evident in the medical treatment of children and adolescents, where there can be an expectation of the child living in one gender, or the other; and where hormone blockers might sometimes be seen as a time-buying measure until the person is old enough to decide whether they want cross-sex hormones. There is often little to no fluidity in medical systems when dealing with young people, and even language reflects an implied gender binary at heart, no matter whether we refer to these children and young people as gender variant, diverse, or creative. The underlying assumption seems to be a deviation from a gender binary norm. Non-binary genders ask us to believe in the possibility that some people have the capacity to simply tell us who they are. A systemic and intersectional framework of gender(s) entails a dynamic understanding of identities as fluid depending on special and temporal locations. Someone might express their non-binary identity more in one context, than another, depending on safety, opportunity, or simply desire.

This approach starts to dismantle several of the structures we have artificially created, in White Western minority cultures, around the gender binary. Medically, cross-sex hormones are seen as masculinising and feminising bodies, usually for the long-term, rather than for manipulating gender traits, within the potential of available chemical compounds. Similarly, surgical interventions often aim to create more masculine or feminine bodies. People with non-binary identities are increasingly seeking to access body modification more as an a la carte, rather than a set menu, challenging how specialist providers are traditionally trained in most countries.

Legally, a non-binary understanding of gender(s) calls us to change the options available to transition—no longer from one end of the spectrum to the other, but potentially to a liminal space, not yet defined in my understanding of legislative rights. This has repercussions not only for individual legal documents, but also for structures regulated according to gender, such as public housing, including shelters; leisure facilities, such as gym and pools; restrooms in public spaces; dormitories in educational institutions; hospitals; and prisons. Besides some *all genders* restrooms and college dormitories, there are currently literally no such spaces explicitly designated for non-binary bodies. It seems reasonable therefore to assume that seeking to create those spaces is another future direction for non-binary genders. As we come to understand gender beyond a binary framework, there is a need to accommodate those genders in a range of public service spaces, if we are to recognise them. Social acceptance and accommodations might increasingly lead to legal and architectural accommodations, especially if non-binary genders can achieve citizenship through legal recognition. In practice, this might mean not segregating bathrooms and other facilities into those for men and for women. The latter is likely to take considerable time, as it seems to be so far outside the current social, legal, and structural organisation of space and relationship within dominant cultures.

If we are not to segregate our shelters, hospitals, prisons, military forces, and restrooms into those for men and those for women, what other systems are available to us? Further, how are we to understand our own humanity given that so much psychological, sociological, cultural, and health knowledge revolves around the polarised dichotomy of men and women (with cisgender status implied)? A non-binary construct of genders calls then for an even deeper structural change in the ways we organise, produce, and reproduce knowledge across a range of disciplines. It invites us to reconsider what we know about being human, about relationships, education, bodies, social roles, and more. When we add in the intersectional aspect of our identities and experiences—as described earlier in this chapter—the picture becomes even more detailed and complex. For example, in public health; are we ready to look at smaller groups, rather than large groups of humans divided by gender first, and then other variables? This means being asked to critically look at what has been considered as the baseline within several disciplines in Anglo-dominant cultures, that is the White, cis, generally (but not exclusively) male, non-disabled, younger, heterosexual, middle-class body. The latter is often what several psychological tests have used to establish their norms; what is represented in medical textbooks; and the basis of several health measures, such as body mass index. Non-binary, intersectional bodies dismantle the very concept of a baseline, since there can be no unit to measure our psyches, bodies, or wellbeing against—if there is no ideal human body, which is a concept that has been promulgated by philosophers, artists, and scientists in Western minority cultures since the heyday of classical Greek culture from Plato to Leonardo da Vinci; from Descartes to Wittgenstein. Without a unit of measurement for humanity, several of our current structures will simply no longer hold.

Brave New World(s)?

This is the point in my writing when I asked myself, what would the world look like if we truly adopted a systemic and intersectional approach to gender(s)? I must admit that there was a long pause of several weeks. Some of the scenarios seemed so futuristic as to border on science fiction. This realisation brought me to another pause to consider why I might be dismissive of science fiction in this chapter? The immediate answer is, of course, that this is a scientific textbook. By definition, science fiction seems to not belong within the realm of non-fiction. However, science fiction has long been the realm of resistance for marginalised identities. As beautifully exemplified in Octavia's Brood (Imarisha & Brown, 2015), science fiction can be the place where visions of the future are explored, especially by those who cannot find room in the context of mainstream, academic knowledge production; and where social justice activists can envision new worlds. In fact, Octavia Butler herself, an African-American science fiction writer, became the first science fiction writer to receive a MacArthur Fellowship, also known as the genius grant. Bringing in Octavia Butler seems relevant in this context given that in her Xenogenesis trilogy (Butler, 2012), she imagines an alien species who include what could be considered a third gender. Non-binary genders are certainly not fictional, and I want to make it clear that this is not what I am implying, and yet imagining a world where non-binary genders are legitimately acknowledged can seem fictional, given the structural repercussions explored above.

In this section of the chapter, I would like to diverge and indulge into a vision of a future where non-binary genders are just genders. What would it look like to be part of a society where gender diversity is the baseline linguistically, culturally, legally, and socially? There is no way to adequately address such a broad question, but here are some potential visions. Children would come into the world as children and no gender would be assigned at birth. Characteristics would be recorded, including genitals, but not gendered. Gender-neutral pronouns would be used until a child could tell us who they are. Their parents and caregivers, as well as the children themselves when a little older, would have access to clothes, accessories, and toys that are not gendered in any specific ways. They would not be divided by gender in daycare, nor would there be assumptions made about their personalities or tendencies based on their genitals. All children would be able to be boisterous, nurturing, express emotions, play, and socialise according to their own desires and not externally imposed norms. At this point, it seems clear that in this utopian world, there would be equitable access to economic, social, and health resources for all as well, and probably no political borders, as the latter seem to significantly interfere with the idea of equitable access. Once children were able to tell us their genders, they would be able to express them freely, including shifting pronouns as desired. If wanted, body modification would be easily available and accessible. Information about options would be part of mainstream education, and the decision process would be collaborative between parents and caregivers, young people, and medical providers. There would be no difference between accessing those services and other medical services. Involvement of any therapists or mental health professionals would be driven by a desire to have space and support to consider the options available and not as a form of gatekeeping or policing of resources.

The variations of genders would be fully integrated in everyday life. This would mean widespread access to all genders restrooms, and no policing of public facilities. There would be no assumed heterosexuality, and therefore no need to segregate people according to a binary idea of gender, given that the multiplicity of genders and sexualities would be accepted as completely human and natural. We would not be able to make assumptions about someone's abilities, personalities, and emotional capacities according to their gender identities, expressions, or roles. There would be a higher proficiency in communicating clearly with one another, and all bodies and intelligences (emotional and sensory, as well as cognitive) would be valued. All architectural structures would be fully accessible. In this utopian world, there would be no misogyny, including trans misogyny, because this could not survive when genders are recognised as multiple and varied; and when there is no assumption that identities, expressions, and roles would align in any particular combination. Such views seem to be incredibly utopian and far fetching. Can I really envision such a world, just starting from a speculation of the future of non-binary gender identities? It seems that I can, in broad strokes, but that the particulars would be impossible to envision through the singular lens of an individual, as they require collective imagination, choices, and actions.

Living with Uncertainty

One of those fundamental choices, and actions, which I am able to take right now, is to practise living with uncertainty. It seems to me that one of the fundamental lies that we have been told is that the world is predictable. Some of the corollaries are, for example, statements such as "if we work hard, we will be rewarded". Data indicate that the working poor work possibly the hardest across the globe, yet earn the least, especially in the USA (DeSante, 2013; Fields, 2012) and other White Western minority societies. As Heraclitus teaches us, the "only constant is change", yet the more privileged we are, the more we believe that we are in control of our destiny, to varying degrees. You might be wondering what this has to do with the future directions of non-binary genders. It seems to me that we are only beginning to understand (again) and to (re)imagine what a world based on gender diversity might look like.

Even though gender diversity has existed as long as human history has been recorded (Feinberg, 1996), inclusion of non-binary genders is likely to look somewhat different than it might have been, because of our different temporal location. If we embrace a systemic and inter-sectional framework of gender(s), it also seems to me that we might one day have more situated knowledge of identities and experiences, including gender. The construct of universal knowledge cannot, in fact, be easily sustained from a systemic and intersectional standpoint, or even from the lens of positioning theory alone. It is likely that different geopolitical social systems might develop different ways of codifying genders, according to linguistic, cultural, and socially situated norms. At the same time, there is no denying that we live in a digital world where Internet access is rapidly increasing, and with it, global connection. What is local is being redefined, and will continue to be redefined as movements, and individuals, connect across space much more easily than ever before—influencing knowledge production and access. Non-binary genders are located within these larger contexts, thriving and evolving within them. This is why I believe it is necessary to become more used to living with uncertainty. The global trend towards mindfulness, and mindfulness-based practices, in White Western minority cultures—albeit commodified through a capitalist framework—seems to reflect people's yearning for holding themselves, each other, and the world, with more open hands. Ultimately, the future trajectories of non-binary genders are likely to be multiple, mutable, and unpredictable. Therefore, I invite you to hold this speculative chapter on future directions, as lightly as it is offered.

Summary

In summary, the future directions of non-binary gender can only be speculated upon. Here are some points made in this chapter:

* If we adopt a systemic and intersectional framework of gender, non-binary gender identities cannot be considered in isolation from other aspects of identity such as race and ethnicity; indigeneity; class; disability; age; religion; and citizenship.
* Non-binary genders blur the polarised dichotomy of trans and cis gender identities. An intersectional view of non-binary genders also challenges trans as an umbrella construct for a range of gender identities.
* In the area of identity labels and politics, one of the potential future directions of non-binary gender identities seems to invite us to truly dismantle cisgenderism; to question the assumed essentialism of masculinity and femininity as natural polarities; to consider our complex, intersectional bodies and lived experiences; and to engage with a different framework of genders altogether.
* A non-binary construct of genders calls for large structural changes, legally, socially, culturally, linguistically, and medically. It also invites a structural change in the ways we organise, produce, and reproduce knowledge across a range of disciplines—inviting us to reconsider what we know about being human, about relationships, education, bodies, social roles, and more; beyond the dichotomy of male/female.
* Non-binary, intersectional bodies dismantle the very concept of a baseline; since there can be no unit to measure our psyches, bodies, or wellbeing against if there is no ideal human body.
* Future directions of non-binary gender are likely to be situated within the paradox of existing and developing—both in specific geopolitical social contexts, and within larger, global digital contexts.

References

Arvin, M., Tuck, E., & Morrill, A. (2013). Decolonizing Feminism: Challenging Connections Between Settler Colonialism and Heteropatriarchy. *Feminist Formations, 25*(1), 8–34.

Boellstorff, T., Cabral, M., Cárdenas, M., Cotten, T., Stanley, E. A., Young, K., et al. (2014). Decolonizing Transgender A Roundtable Discussion. *TSQ: Transgender Studies Quarterly, 1*(3), 419–439.

Butler, O. E. (2012). *Lilith's Brood: Dawn, Adulthood Rites, and Imago*. New York: Open Road Media.

Cho, S., Crenshaw, K. W., & McCall, L. (2013). Toward a Field of Intersectionality Studies: Theory, Applications, and Praxis. *Signs, 38*(4), 785–810.

Coleman, E., Bockting, W., Botzer, M., Cohen-Kettenis, P., DeCuypere, G., Feldman, J., et al. (2012). Standards of Care for the Health of Transsexual, Transgender, and Gender-nonconforming People, version 7. *International Journal of Transgenderism, 13*(4), 165–232.

Crenshaw, K. (1991). Mapping the Margins: Intersectionality, Identity Politics, and Violence Against Women of Color. *Stanford Law Review, 43*(6), 1241–1299.

Currah, P. (2006). Gender Pluralisms Under the Transgender Umbrella. *Transgender rights*, 3–31.

DeSante, C. D. (2013). Working Twice as Hard to get Half as Far: Race, Work Ethic, and America's Deserving Poor. *American Journal of Political Science, 57*(2), 342–356.

Dutta, A., & Roy, R. (2014). Decolonizing Transgender in India Some Reflections. *TSQ: Transgender Studies Quarterly, 1*(3), 320–337.

Feinberg, L. (1996). *Transgender Warriors: Making History from Joan of Arc to Dennis Rodman*. Boston, MA: Beacon Press.

Fields, G. S. (2012). *Working Hard, Working Poor: A Global Journey*. New York: OUP.

Harré, R., & Van Langenhove, L. (Eds.). (1998). *Positioning Theory: Moral Contexts of International Action*. Hoboken, NJ: Wiley-Blackwell.

Harrison, J., Grant, J., & Herman, J. L. (2012). A Gender Not Listed Here: Genderqueers, Gender Rebels, and Otherwise in the National Transgender Discrimination Survey. *LGBTQ Public Policy Journal at the Harvard Kennedy School, 2*(1), 13.

Iantaffi, A., & Bockting, W. O. (2011). Views from Both Sides of the Bridge? Gender, Sexual Legitimacy and Transgender People's Experiences of Relationships. *Culture, Health & Sexuality, 13*(3), 355–370.

Iantaffi, A. (2015). Gender and Sexual Legitimacy. *Current Sexual Health Reports, 7*(2), 103–107.

Imarisha, W., & Brown, A. M. (2015). *Octavia's Brood: Science Fiction Stories from Social Justice Movements.* Oakland, CA: AK Press and the Institute for Anarchist Studies.

Irving, D. (2008). Normalized Transgressions: Legitimizing the Transsexual Body as Productive. *Radical History Review, 100,* 38.

King, M., Smith, A., & Gracey, M. (2009). Indigenous Health Part 2: The Underlying Causes of the Health Gap. *The Lancet, 374*(9683), 76–85.

Lamble, S. (2008). Retelling Racialized Violence, Remaking White Innocence: The Politics of Interlocking Oppressions in Transgender Day of Remembrance. *Sexuality Research & Social Policy, 5*(1), 24–42.

Richards, C., Barker, M., Lenihan, P., & Iantaffi, A. (2014). Who Watches the Watchmen? A Critical Perspective on the Theorization of Trans People and Clinicians. *Feminism & Psychology, 24*(2), 248–258. doi:10.1177/0959353514526220.

Richards, C., Bouman, W. P., Seal, L., Barker, M. J., Nieder, T. O., & T'Sjoen, G. (2016). Non-binary or Genderqueer Genders. *International Review of Psychiatry, 28*(1), 95–102.

Robinson, M. (2012). Two-Spirited Sexuality and White Universality. *Plural Space, Postcolonial Networks: Pursuing Global Justice Together.* Retrieved January 6, 2014, from http://postcolonialnetworks.com/2012/06/02/two-spirited/

Steinmetz, K.. (2014, May 29). The transgender tipping point. *Time.*

Wyer, M., Barbercheck, M., Cookmeyer, D., Ozturk, H., & Wayne, M. (2013). *Women, Science, and Technology: A Reader in Feminist Science Studies.* Abingdon, UK: Routledge.

Index[1]

[1] Note: Page numbers followed by "n" denote notes.

© The Author(s) 2017
C. Richards et al. (eds.), *Genderqueer and Non-Binary Genders*, Critical and Applied
Approaches in Sexuality, Gender and Identity, DOI 10.1057/978-1-137-51053-2

Made in the USA
Middletown, DE
11 July 2018